Neuroscience Mind Maps

A 'go-to' book to master the complex mechanisms of the brain

Swapnil Paralikar
DC Mathangi

notionpress.com

INDIA • SINGAPORE • MALAYSIA

ISBN 979-8-89277-627-1

Dedicated

To my parents Alka Paralikar and Dr. Jagdish Paralikar

For their compassion and care and for instilling in me the love of books And to my students

Who inspired me to hone my skills at teaching

Swapnil Paralikar

To my parents and to my students

DC Mathangi

Contents

Authors

Dr. Swapnil Paralikar
MD, FAIMER (CMC Ludhiana),ACME
Associate Professor, Department of Physiology
Government Medical College, Bhavnagar
Bhavnagar, Gujarat-364002. INDIA.
E-mail :drsparalikar@gmail.com –
M- 9879119740

Dr. D C Mathangi
Professor and Head
Department of Mind Body Medicine and Lifestyle Sciences
Sri Ramachandra Institute of Higher Education and Research, Porur,
Chennai-60016. INDIA
E-mail : dcmathangi@gmail.com
M- 9940635874

Contributors

1. **Dr. K Soundariya**
   Professor,
   Department of Physiology
   Sri ManakulaVinayanagar Medical College and Hospital
   Puducherry 605107 India.
   drsoundariya@gmail.com

2. **Dr. RituparnaBarooah**
   Professor and Head Department of Physiology
   Northeastern Indira Gandhi Institute of Health Sciences and Medical Sciences
   Shillong 793018
   Meghalaya, India
   drrituparnabarooah@gmail.com

3. **Dr. Lata Bukhar**
   Associate Professor Department of Physiology SVNGMC
   Yavatmal, Maharashtra, India.
   latabuktar@gmail.com

4. **Dr.MadhulikaMonga**
   Professor
   Lady Hardinge Medical College
   New Delhi 110 001.
   India.
   madhulika.monga@gmail.com

5. **Dr.Thejwasni KO**
   Professor and Head Department of Physiology,
   Sri Siddhartha Institute of Medical Sciences and Research Centre,
   T-Begur, Bangalore Rural, 562123
   thejaswiniko78@gmail.com

Preface

"Everything should be made as simple as possible, but not simpler." - Albert Einstein

India is in the throes of major curricular change. A new Competency driven curriculum has been rolled out by the National Medical Commission in 2019.

Neuroscience is the holy grail for medical students. Most students can understand and apply the concepts of the other organ systems after going through the traditional textbooks. Neuroscience offers enormous challenges because of its intricacy . Indeed , many concepts in this domain are being unravelled as of today . This makes the task of mastering Neuroscience even more daunting.

The aim of this book is to enable the medical students to understand the fundamentals of Neuroscience and revise them quickly. Physiology is the basis of clinical medicine. Hence, the Mind Maps are organized such that Physiology is linked aptly with the relevant aspects of clinical medicine. This book is organized based on the new Competency Based Medical Education (CBME) curriculum rolled out by the NMC. Each Mind Map covers the functional anatomy (wherever necessary), has a lucid explanation of the concepts of physiology, and highlights the relevant molecular and clinical aspects. Only those molecular aspects have been delineated which are the targets of pharmacological agents or form the basis for understanding the mechanisms of disease. The maps focus on fostering a robust understanding of physiology that may facilitate better and quick recall. Mind Maps enable the student to form a visuo-spatial memory of the topic. This template harnesses the evidence from cognitive psychology. Visuo-spatial memory coupled with spaced repetition and recall is the recipe for mastering a concept.

Lastly, we have made an honest endeavour to be as accurate as possible. Physiology is a dynamic branch, with Neuroscience evolving at a brisker pace. We welcome suggestions from the students and teachers regarding room for improvement . We sincerely hope that students embrace learning through Mind Maps and apply it in other subjects and spheres of life, as well.

Swapnil Paralikar

DC Mathangi

(5th October 2023)

Acknowledgement to

Dr. Sanjay Bedi and MEU India

For introducing us to the world of mind maps and for being there throughout the writing of this book

&

Dr. Prasan Bhandari

For teaching us the art of making mind maps

Curtain Raiser

The Concept of Mind Mapping

Swapnil Paralikar

Introduction:

Each day 3,85,000 babies are born around the world. Within a span of two months, these babies will begin to recognize their mother's face. The latter forms an anchor for navigating the world. Memories of other aspects of the baby's world are formed with regards to the mother's face. Thus, the baby has a visual memory and spatial relationship with each object with regards to the mother.

American psychologist Tony Buzan pioneered a technique called Mind Mapping. He developed the technique to facilitate taking notes in lectures before he went on to apply his seemingly innocuous creation in all spheres of his life. Mind Mapping harnesses the evidence from cognitive psychology regarding learning. Today, Buzan's Mind Mapping technique is immensely popular worldwide.

Though Tony Buzan is the modern 'guru' of Mind Maps, he himself does not take credit of being the pioneer of Mind Maps. In his seminal book, 'Mind Map Mastery', Buzan has cited a number of scholars who had used this technique centuries ago. When Charles Darwin proclaimed his theory of evolution to the world, he intuitively drew his 'tree of life' like a Mind Map. The versatile and maverick painter, Leonardo de Vinci, made numerous drawings resembling Mind Maps. Thus,learning, and creative expression through Mind Maps has enamoured mankind since ages.

Students in various disciplines learn by memorizing facts and then decipher the concept. Now, a large body of evidence has been published on 'smart' study strategies. Among these, Barbara Oakley's technique of spaced repetition and active recall has gained prominence. Mind Maps are a repertoire among this armament of study techniques. However, textbooks with Mind Maps are scanty. The education community has not yet harnessed the power of this simple, yet elegant and holistic strategy to foster better learning.

What are Mind Maps?

A Mind Map is a colourful visual diagram used to capture information. It has three essential elements:

i. A central idea/image

ii. Branches radiating out from the central image.

iii. A single key word/idea/image on each branch

How to make a Mind Map?

The following are the seven steps to make a 'good' Mind Map.

Step 1

Take a sheet of paper (A4 size), and place it in landscape mode (horizontally).

Write a central idea/word or draw a colourful image in the centre.

For the sake of simplicity, we will be making a Mind Map on cell organelles.

Step 2

Pick a distinct colour and draw a branch radiating from the centre.

Step 3

The branch should be labelled with the name of a cell organelle. The thickness of the branch should be ideally proportional to the relative importance of the cell organelle.

Step 4

Draw secondary level shoots from the main branch e.g., for mitochondria, the secondary level shoots could be structure, function and applied aspects.

Step 5

Pick another color and draw another main branch and so on.

Step 6

After drawing all the main branches, you should follow steps 2 and 3.

Step 7

You may draw arrows or connections connecting the main branches. This highlights the relationship between objects.

Why should we practice and use Mind Mapping?

First and foremost, the reader needs to be acquainted with some fundamentals of cognitive neuroscience. Learning is the ability to alter behaviour based on past experiences. Memory is the retention and storage of new information. Learning cannot occur without memory; on the other hand, memory depends on learning for its very existence. Thus, learning and memory are opposite, yet complementary sides of the same coin.

There are two broad categories of memory: Declarative and Non-Declarative. The latter involves skills, habits, and conditioned reflexes. In cognitive neuroscience, Declarative Memory is divided into Semantic Memory and Episodic Memory. Semantic Memory is the memory for facts, words, rules, language. It forms a major chunk of our memory. Episodic memory is the memory of events/episodes. For examples, knowing that India won the 2011 Men's Cricket World Cup is Semantic Memory. On the other hand, remembering what one was doing or who were the other people around, when Dhoni hit the winning six, is Episodic Memory.

A large body of evidence suggests the role of the medial temporal lobe in forming declarative memories. The hippocampus (=sea horse) is ensconced within this medial temporal lobe. The classic case of HM (Henry Molaison) affords enough evidence regarding the role of the hippocampus in forming declarative memory. HM lost all ability to form new memories after his medial temporal lobe was removed in his twenties to treat his epileptic seizures.

John o Keefe at the University College, London and Lynn Nadel at the University of Arizona proposed the **cognitive mapping theory** to explain the role of the hippocampus in memory. According to this theory, the hippocampus has *place cells* which fire when the animal is at a particular place in relation to its local environment. London taxi drivers with several years of experience had much larger hippocampi compared to controls, a testimony to the cognitive mapping theory.

In the 1990s, Howard Eichenbaum at Boston University and Neal Cohen at the University of Illinois, proposed **a relational memory theory**. According to this theory, the hippocampus does not mediate the representation of space as such, but represents a memory space. Thus, the relationships between objects are coded by the conjunction of overlapping cues. Mind Maps provide a visuo-spatial relationship between related ideas or concepts. Hence, they harness the prowess of these theories of cognitive neuroscience to facilitate the formation of robust declarative memory leading thereafter to the desired level of recall. In addition, colours and images harness the power of the representational hemisphere and words that of the categorical hemisphere. Mind Maps are thus, the epitome of learning through sound cognitive neuroscience. No wonder, it is a wonderful tool to foster learning and memory of any concept.

To sum up, a mind map is a colorful diagram used to depict concepts in any sphere of life. They harness the power of cognitive neuroscience (cognitive mapping theory and relational memory theory), and the unique strengths of each hemisphere of the cerebral cortex. Thus, they facilitate better learning and optimum recall.

References:

1. Buzan T. Mind map mastery: The complete guide to learning and using the most powerful thinking tool in the universe. Watkins Media Limited; 2018 Mar 13.
2. Purves D, Cabeza R, Huettel SA, LaBar KS, Platt ML, Woldorff MG, Brannon EM. Cognitive neuroscience. Sunderland: Sinauer Associates, Inc; 2008.

Mind Maps have been designed on computer software by

Dr. Swapnil Paralikar

SECTION I

PERIPHERAL NERVOUS SYSTEM

1. Organization of the Nervous System

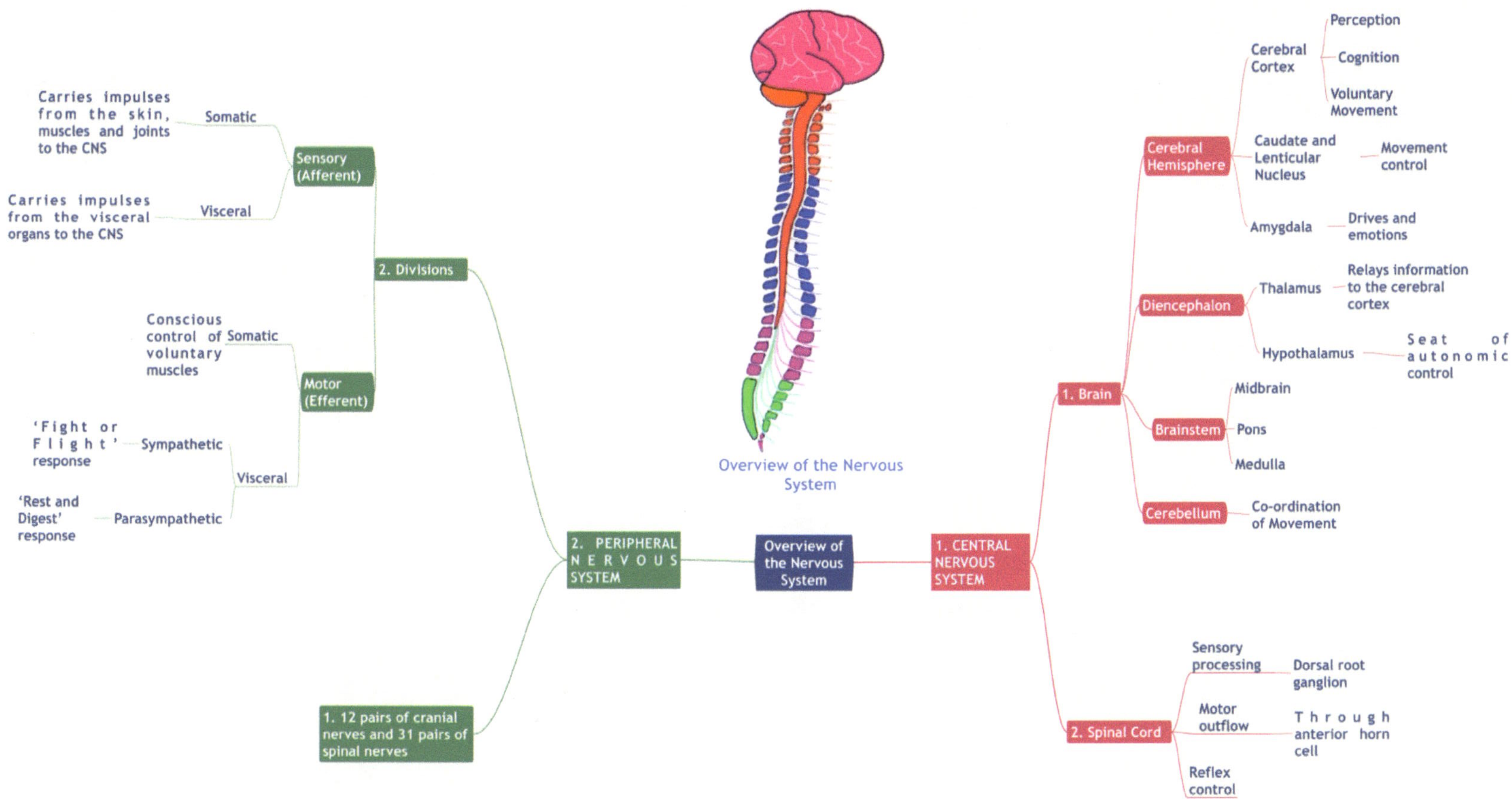

DC Mathangi

2. Neuron

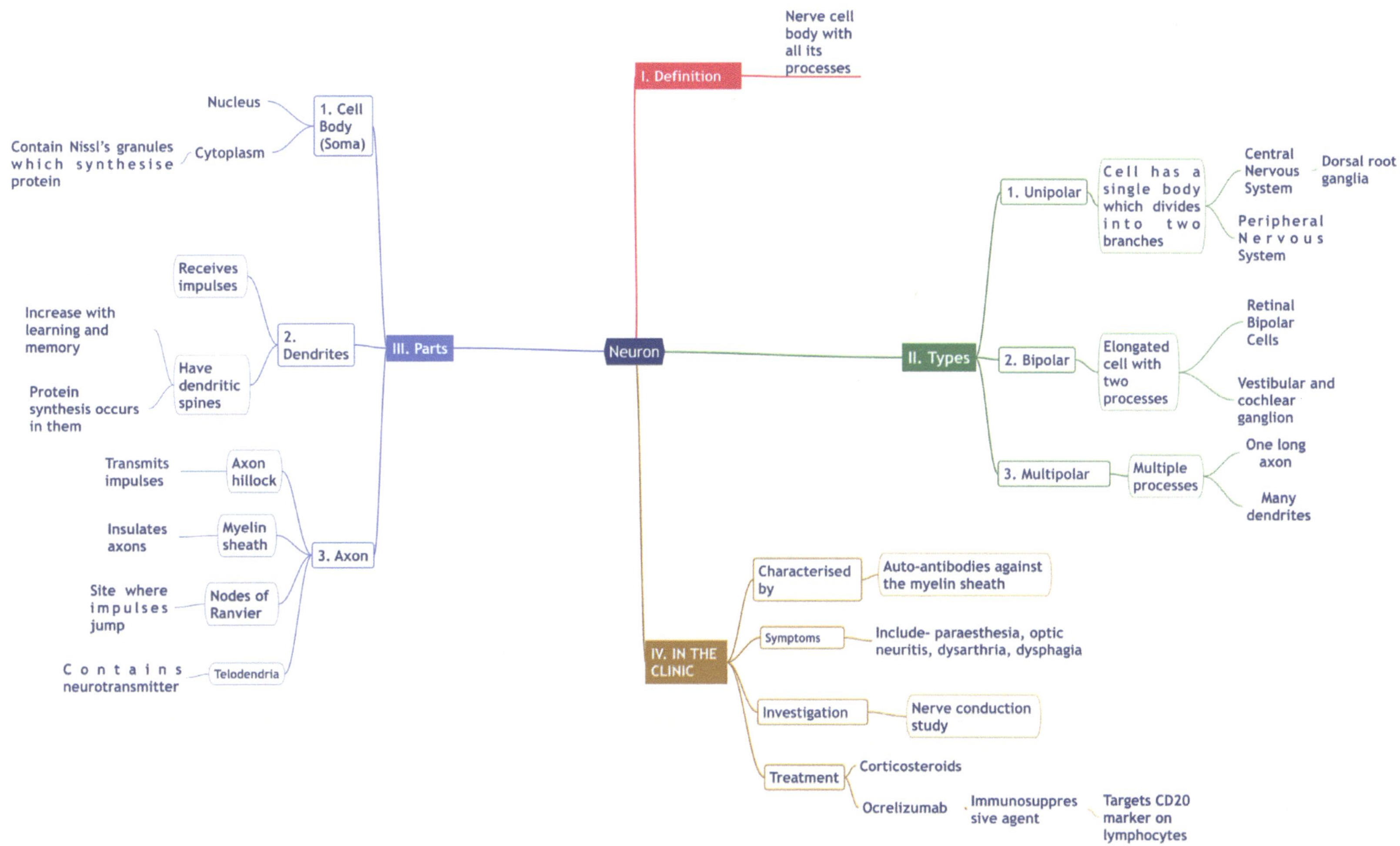

Swapnil Paralikar

3. Neuroglia

- Neuroglia
  - 1. Astrocytes
    - Contribute to homeostasis
      - 1. Blood Brain Barrier
        - Inductive interaction
          - Perivascular end feet
          - CNS capillaries
      - 2. Energy metabolism
        - Store glycogen and lactate
      - 3. Glutamate-glutamine cycle
        - Helps take up glutamate and converted to glutamine
          - Recycled to glutamate
      - 4. Potassium Homeostasis
        - Buffers potassium in the extra-cellular fluid
  - 2. Oligodendrocytes
    - Form myelin sheath in the CNS
  - 3. Schwann Cells
    - Form myelin sheath in the PNS
  - 4. Microglia
    - Phagocytic cells of the CNS

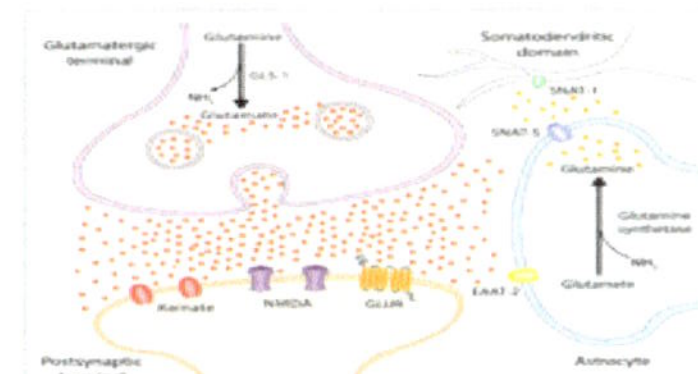
Glutamate Glutamine cycle

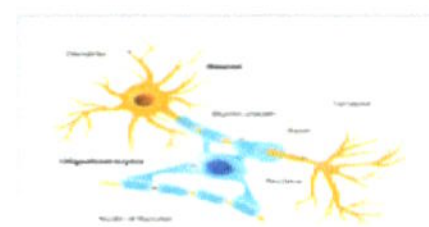
Oligodendrocytes

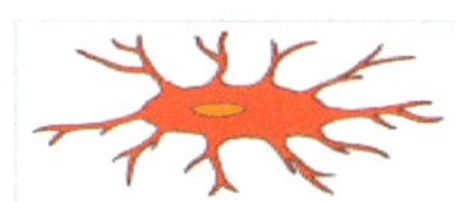
Microglia

Swapnil Paralikar

4. Synapse

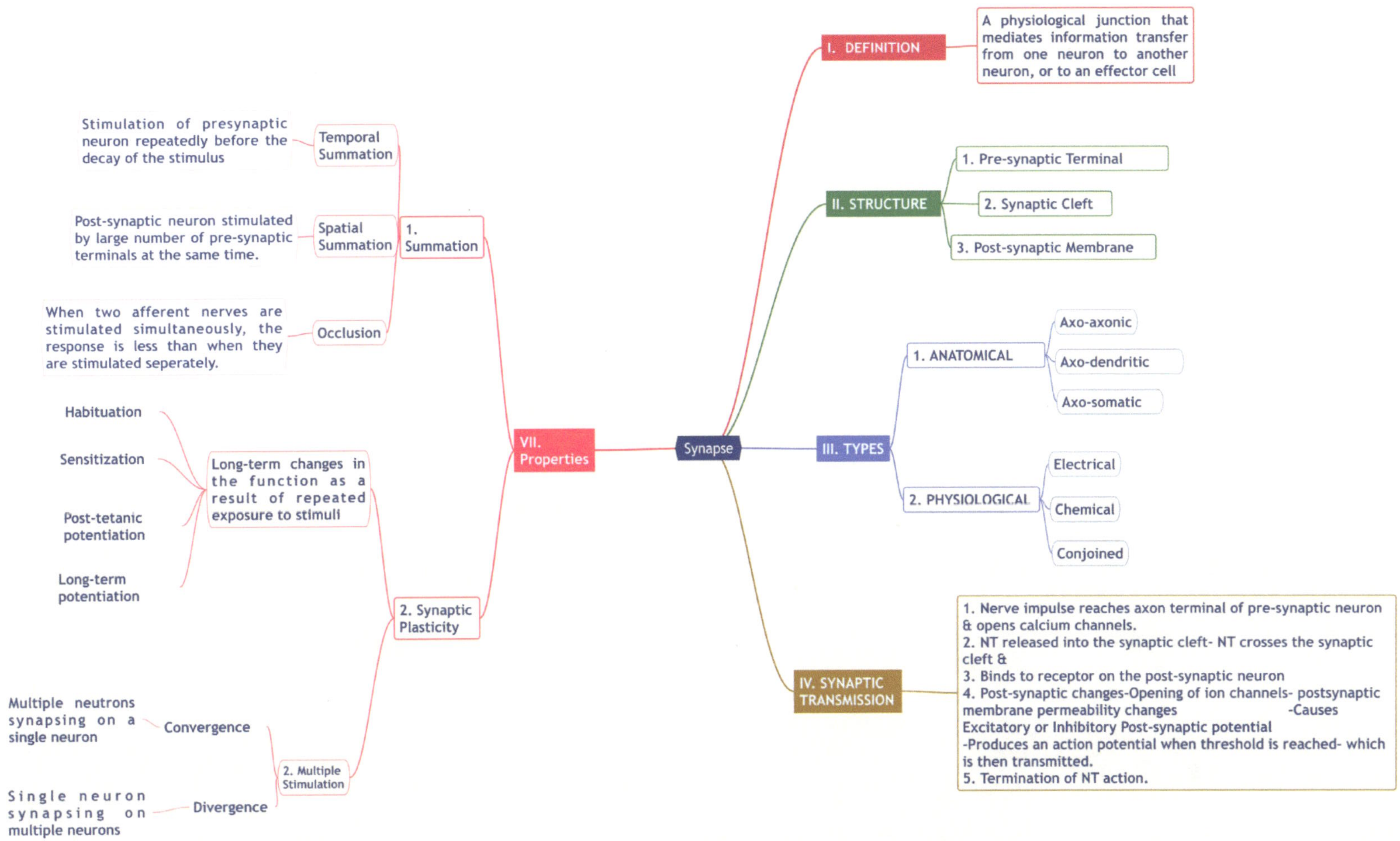

DC Mathangi

5. Receptors

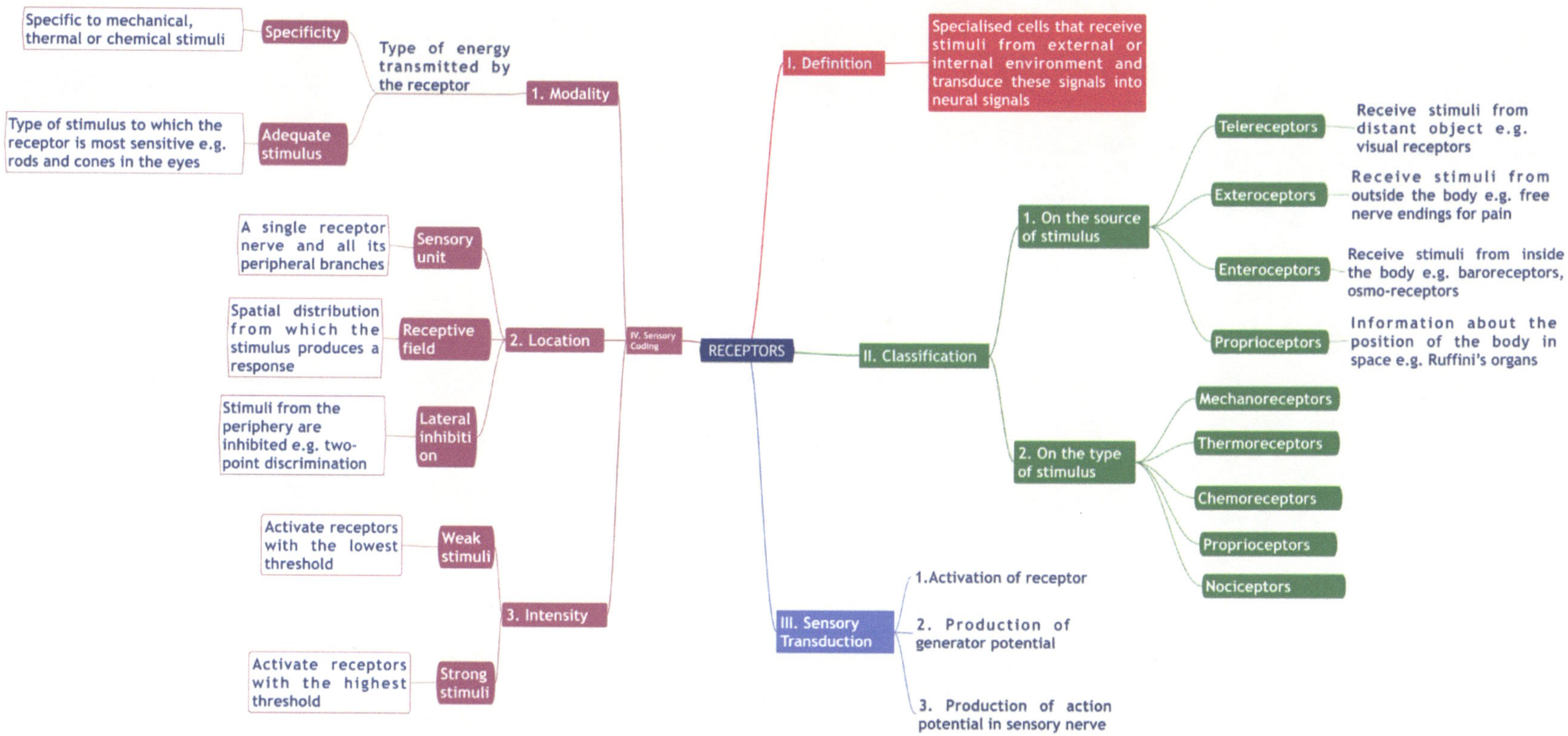

DC Mathangi

6. Reflexes-I

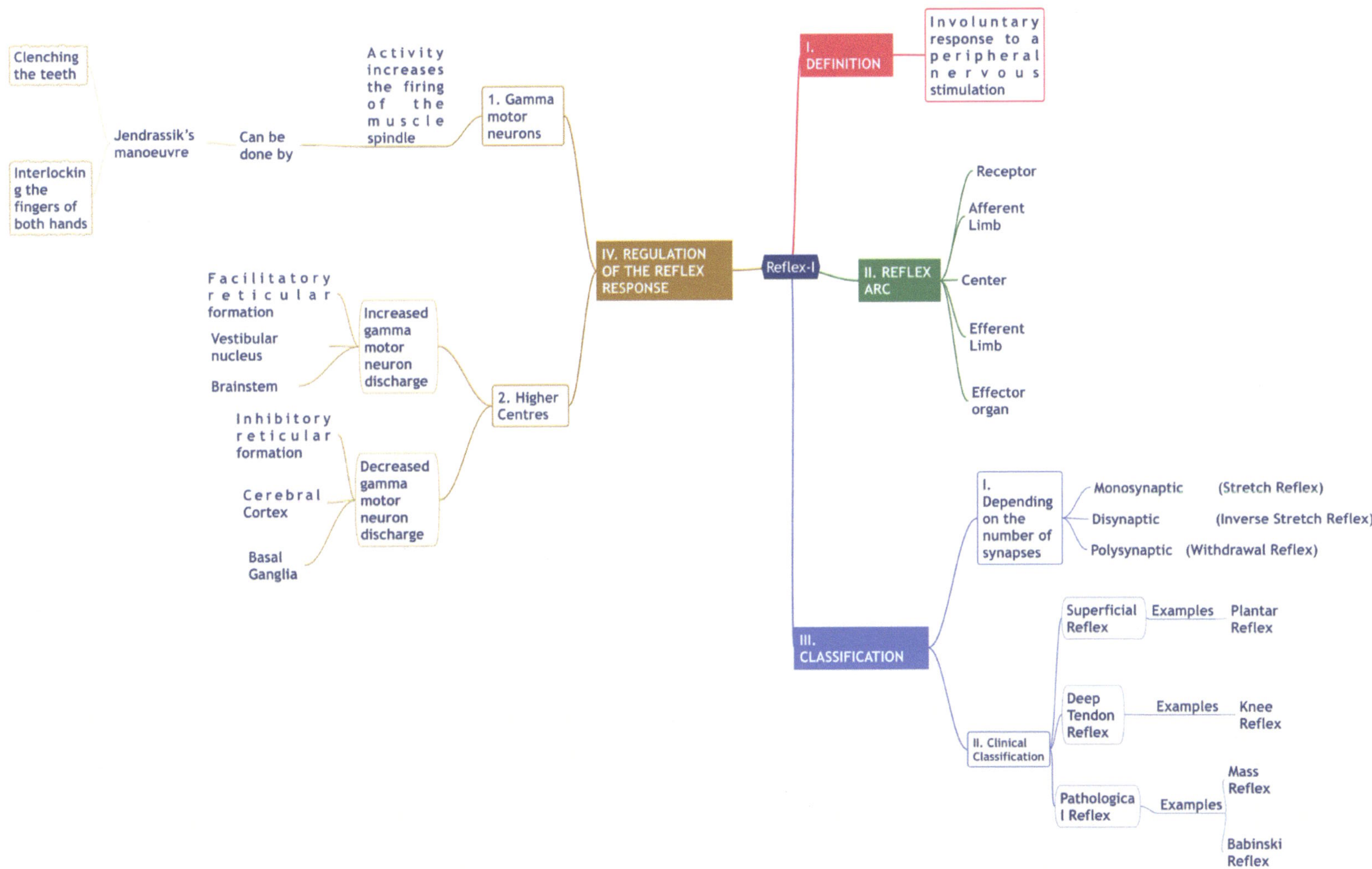

K S Soundariya

7. Reflexes-II

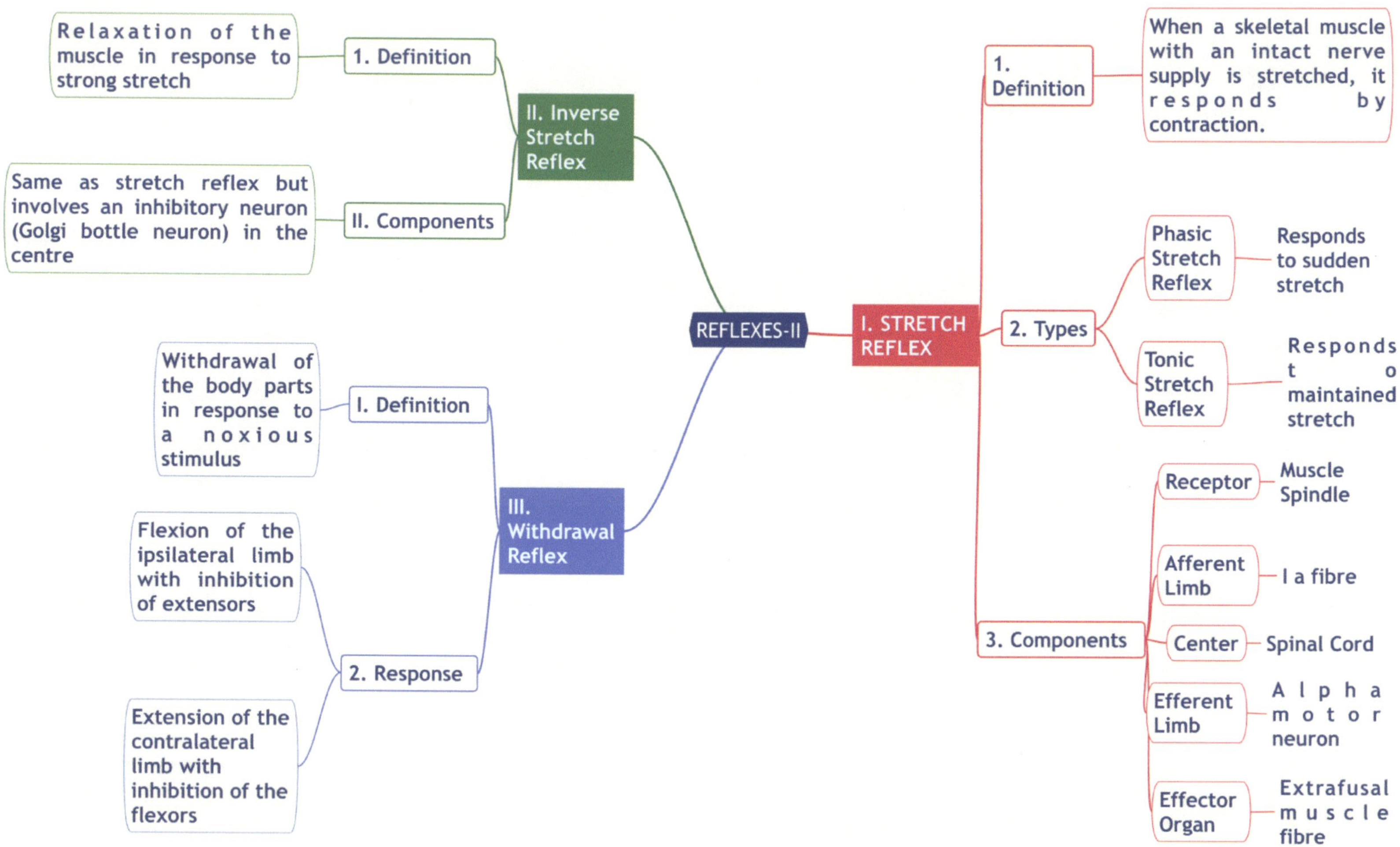

Swapnil Paralikar

8. Physiology of Pain-I

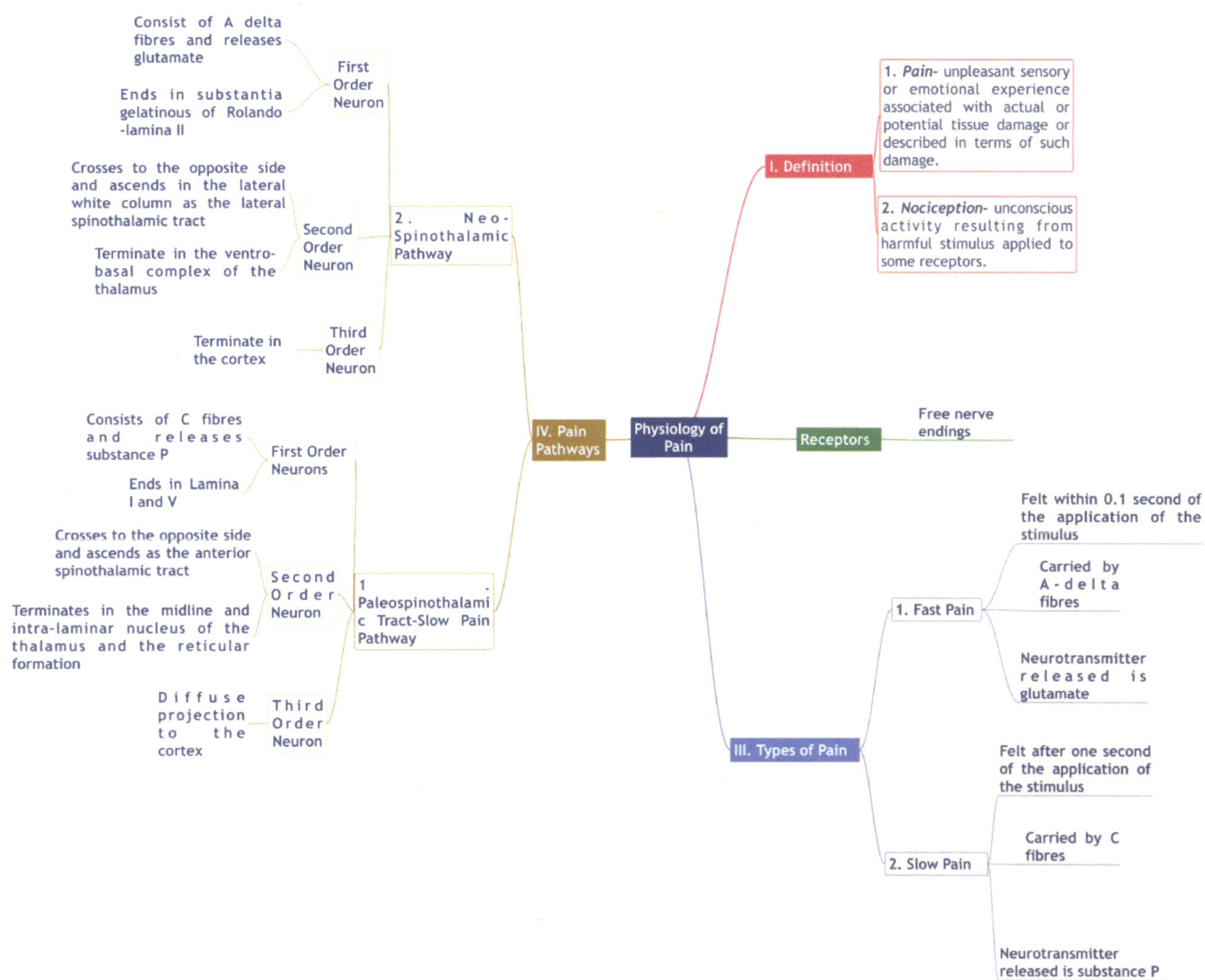

K S Soundariya

9. Physiology of Pain-II-Applied Physiology of Pain

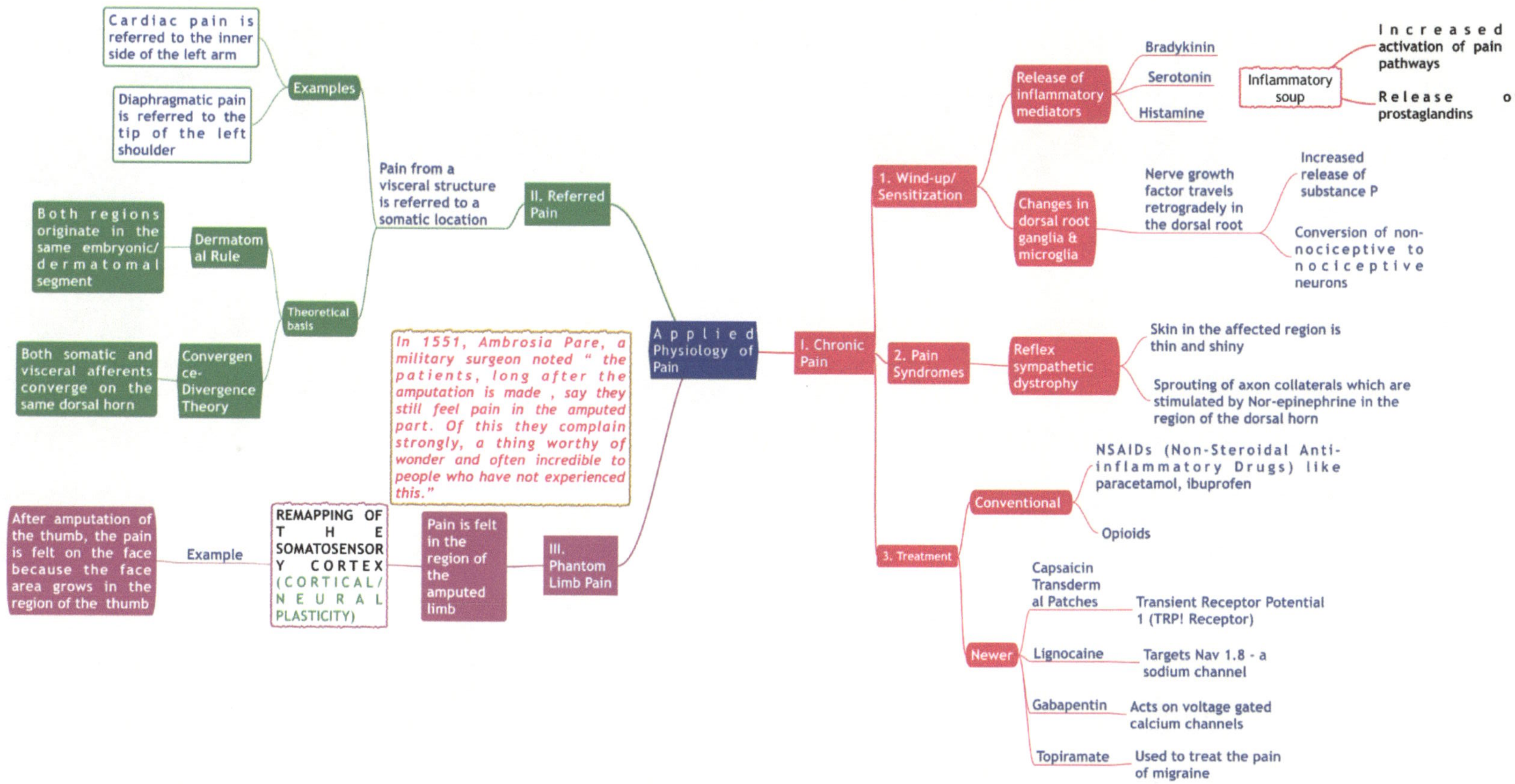

Swapnil Paralikar

10. Analgesia System

- **Analgesia System**
  - I. Endogenous Pain Inhibiting System
    - 1. Gate control theory of Pain
      - Stimulation of large diameter touch fibres inhibits pain sensation in the dorsal horn by lateral inhibition
    - 2. Supra-spinal system
      - Fibres from the peri-aqueductal region and peri-ventricular region of the brain stem release OPIATES and inhibit pain sensation
        - Opiates
          - Act pre-synaptically by decreasing calcium influx
          - Act post-synaptically by increasing potassium conductance and causing hyperpolarization
  - II. Endogenous Pain Inhibitors
    - 1. Opiod Peptides
      - Endorphins
        - Supra-spinal and spinal anaesthesia
        - Produce euphoria- 'runner's high'
        - *Adverse reaction*
          - Constipation
          - Sedation
          - Miosis
    - 2. Cannabinoids
      - ANANDIMIDE
        - CB1 receptors
          - Produce euphoria
        - CB2 receptors
          - Act on activated microglia and reduce the inflammatory response to neuropathic pain
  - III. Stress induced analgesia
    - Soldiers released in the heat of the battle feel little/no pain
      - Due to the release of
        - OPIATES

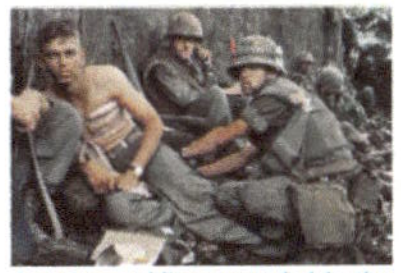

American soldiers wounded in the Vietnam war felt little or no pain during battle due to the release of opiods

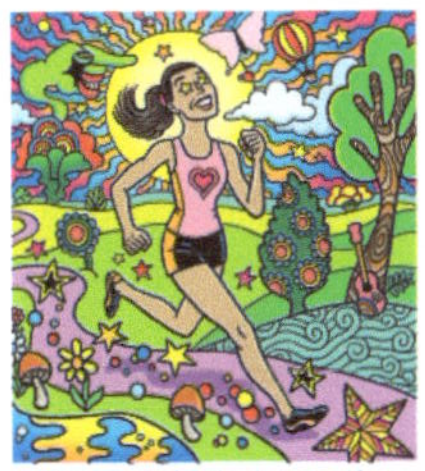

Runner's high due to the release of endogenous opioids (endorphins)

Swapnil Paralikar

11. Ascending Tracts-I- Dorsal Column Medial Lemniscal System

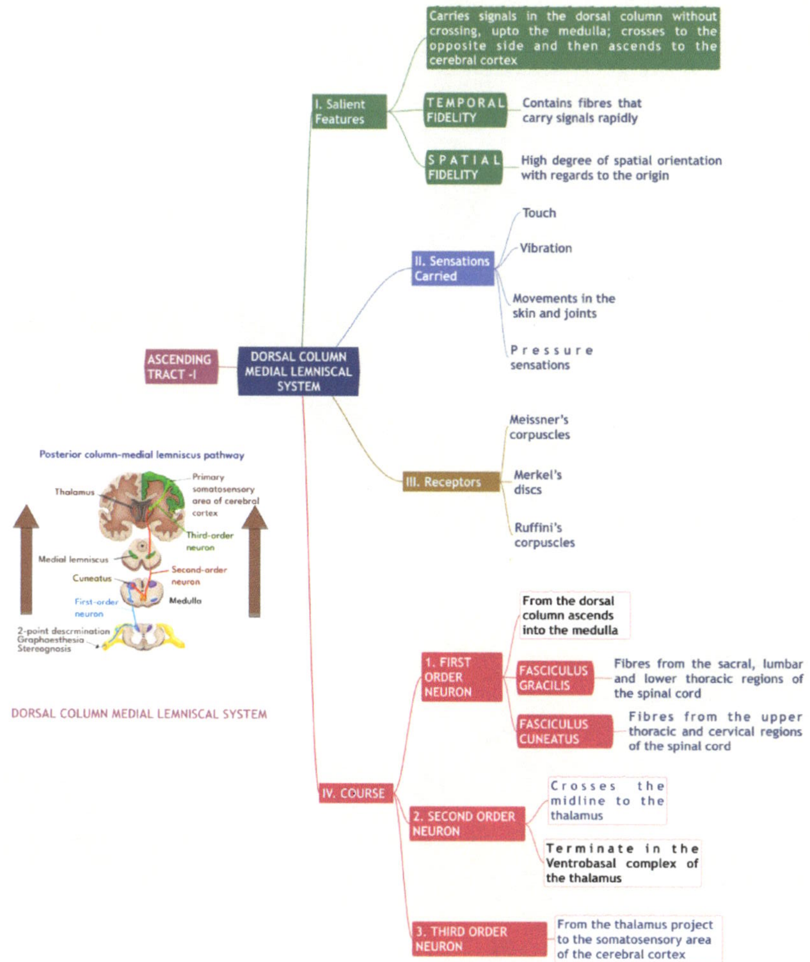

Lata Bukhar & Swapnil Paralikar

12. Ascending Tracts-II-Anterolateral System

ASCENDING TRACTS-II → **Anterolateral System**

- **I. Salient Features**
  - While carrying sensory signals to the central nervous system, immediately crosses to the opposite side at the spinal cord; ascends through the anterior and lateral white columns
  - Transmits a broad spectrum of sensory modalities
- **II. Sensations carried**
  - Thermoceptive sensations
    - Warmth
    - Cold
  - Pain
  - Tickle and itch
  - Sexual sensations
- **III. Receptors**
  - Free nerve endings
- **IV. Course**
  - **1. First Order Neurons**
    - From the receptor to the laminae of the dorsal horn
  - **2. Second Order Neurons**
    - Crosses to the opposite side and ascends in the anterior white column as the ANTERIOR SPINO-THALAMIC TRACT
    - Crosses to the opposite side and ascends in the lateral white column as the LATERAL SPINO-THALAMIC TRACT
    - Terminates in the Ventro-basal complex and the intra-laminar nucleus of the thalamus
  - **3. Third Order Neurons**
    - From the thalamus projects to the somatosensory cortex

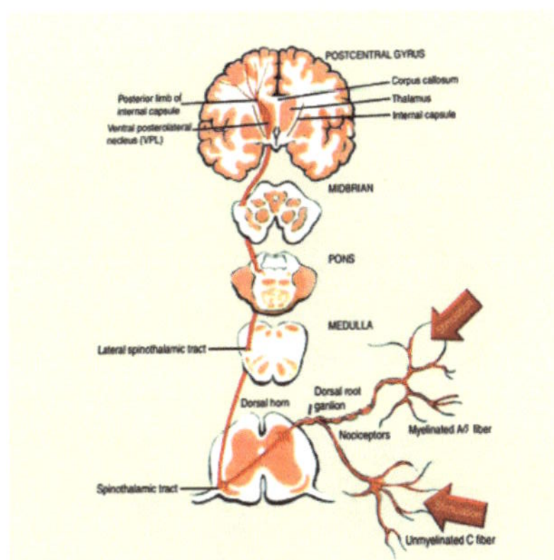

THE ANTERO-LATERAL SYSTEM: SPINO-THALAMIC TRACTS

13. Corticospinal Tracts

- **Corticospinal Tract**
  - Connects the cerebral cortex to the spinal motor neurons
    - Controls the voluntary movement of the torso and the upper and lower limbs
  - **Origin**
    - Cerebral Motor Cortex (30%)
    - Premotor Cortex (30%)
    - Somatosensory Cortex I and II (40%)
  - **Course**
    - Converge towards the brainstem as a corona radiate to reach the internal capsule
    - Passes via the midbrain (medial 3/5th) to the pons
    - Tract is broken as a series of bundles by nuclei pontis to the medulla
    - Scattered bundles re-unite and enter the medulla-form the thick anterior portion of the medulla - PYRAMIDS
  - **Motor Decussation**
    - 80% crosses and decussates as the Lateral Cortico-spinal Tract
    - 20% uncrossed fibres descend as the Anterior Cortico-spinal Tract
  - **Termination**
    - Lateral Cortico-spinal Tract
      - Terminate in internuncial neurons in grey matter in the anterior horn of the spinal cord
    - Anterior Cortico-spinal Tract
      - Crosses at the spinal level
        - Controls the axial movement of the head and trunks
  - **Functions**
    - Controls voluntary movements
    - Controls superficial reflexes
    - Controls muscle tone
  - **Lesions**
    - Upper motor neuron type of paralysis

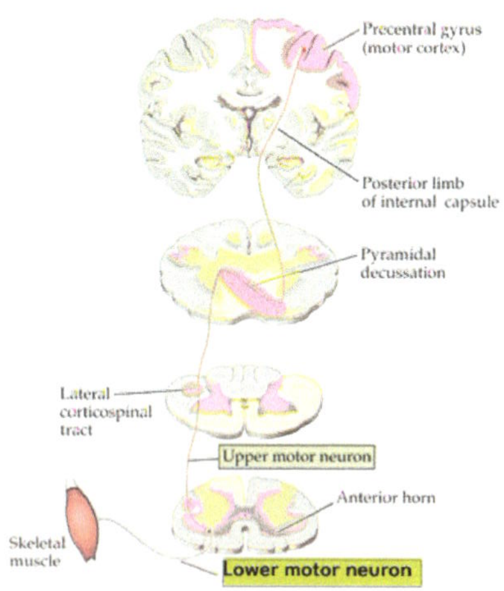

Lateral Cortico-spinal Tract

DC Mathangi

14. Extra-pyramidal Tracts

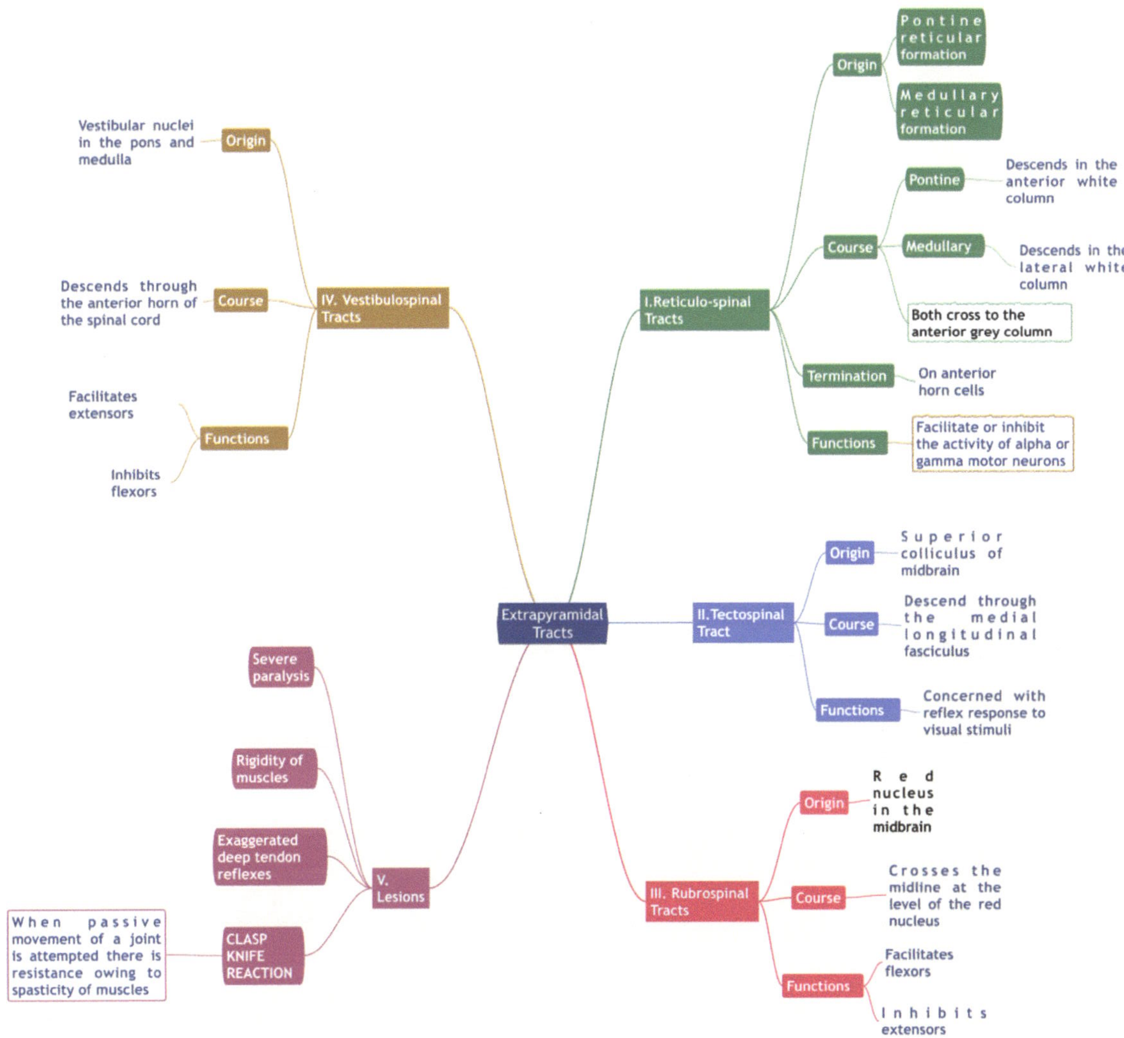

Swapnil Paralikar

15. Lesions of Motor Tracts

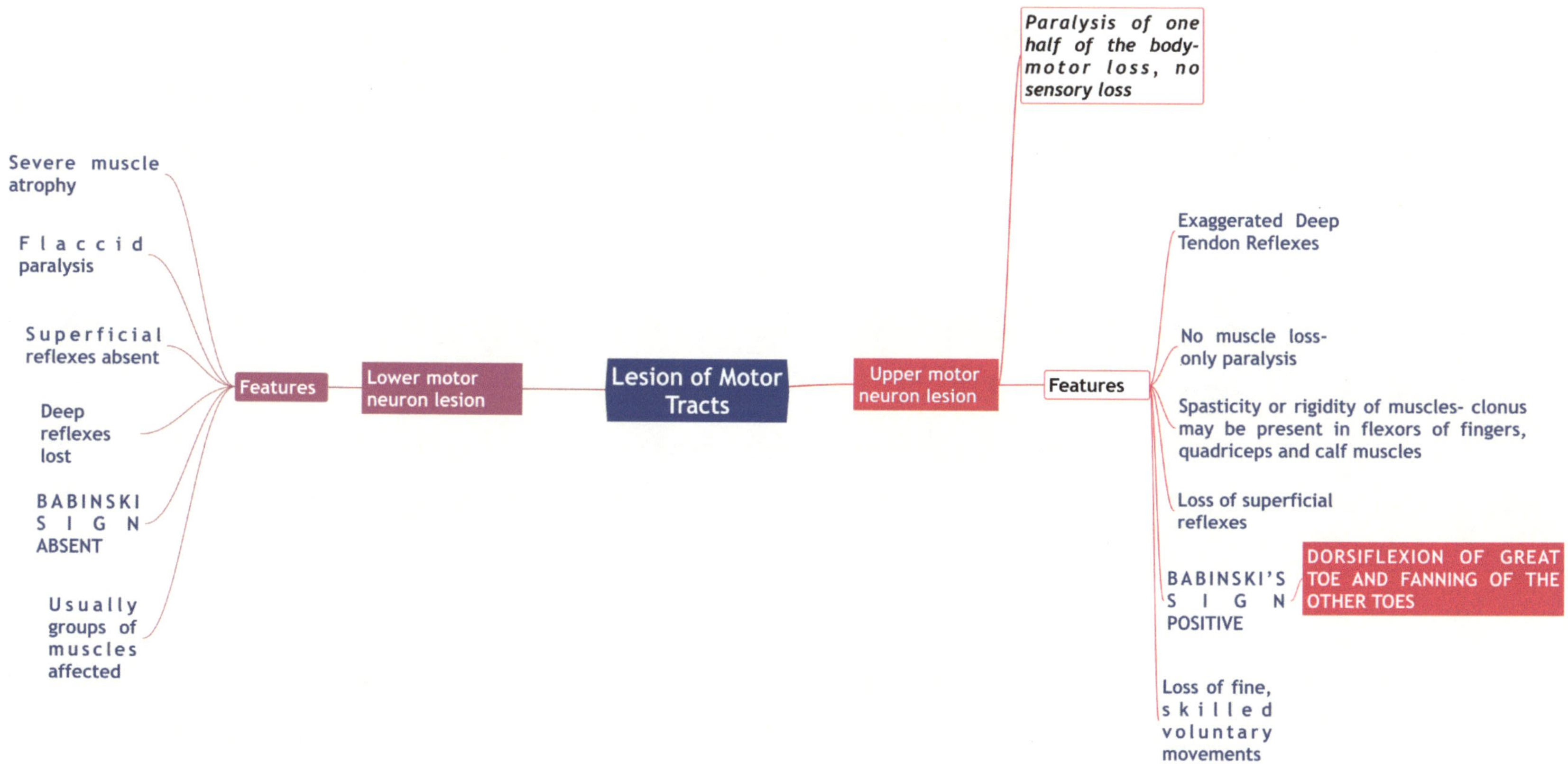

DC Mathangi

16. Muscle Tone

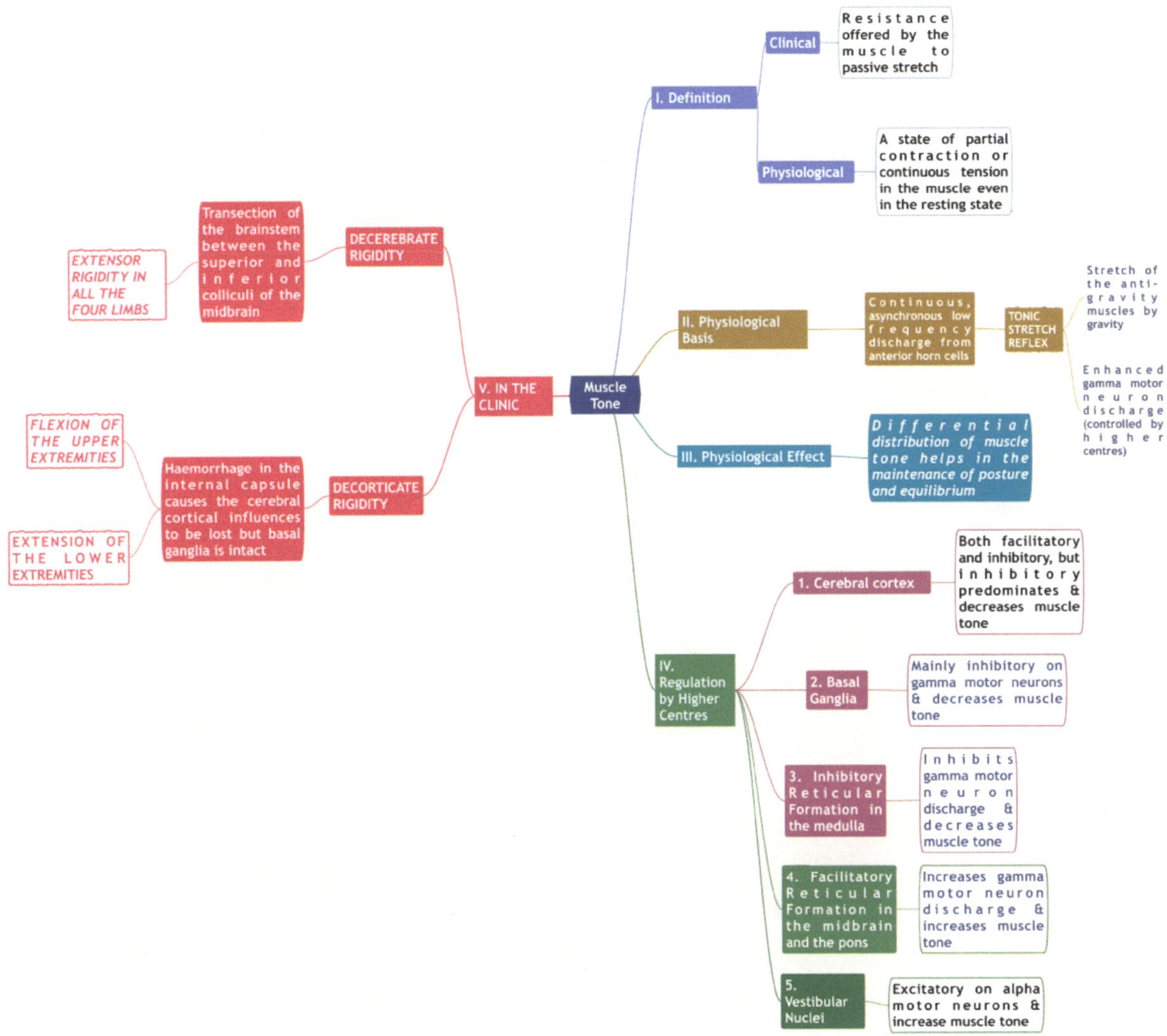

K S Soundariya

17. Vestibular Apparatus

Vestibular Apparatus

- **I. Components**
  - **Semicircular canals**
    - Angular acceleration of the head
    - Rotation of the head
  - **Saccule and utricle**
    - Linear acceleration of the head
    - Translational motion
    - Gravity (and by extension head tilt)
      - Saccule- sagittal
      - Utricle- horizontal

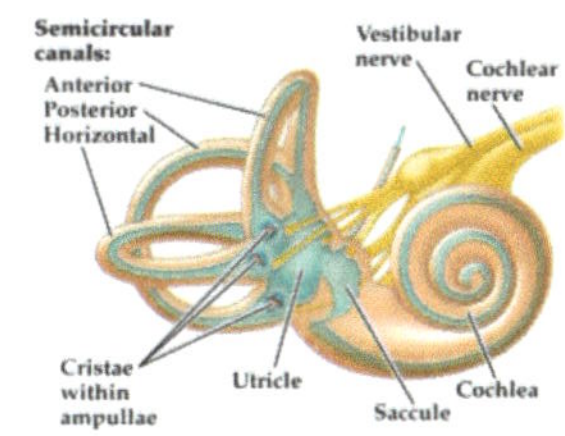

Vestibular Apparatus

- **II. Specialised Receptors**
  - **Crista ampullaris**
  - **Macula**
    - Two types of sensory structures: KINOCILIUM & stereocilia
      - Depolarized: bending of stereo cilia towards the kinocilium
      - Hyperpolarized: bending of stereo cilia away from the kinocilium

- **III. Vestibular Pathway**
  - **1. Overview**
    - VIII cranial nerve to vestibular nuclei
    - Vestibular nuclei make connections with cranial nuclei associated with ocular movements (III, IV and VI) and cerebellum
  - **2. Detailed Pathway**
    - - Receptors: Crista Ampullaris, Macula
      -1st order neurons: Afferent fibres from hair cells to dendrites of bipolar cells
    - - Afferents : vestibular apparatus; inhibitory fibres from cerebellum and cerebrum
      - Efferents :
      Vestibulo-spinal tract
      Vestibulo-ocular tract
      Vestibuloreticulo-spinal tract
      Vestibulo-rubrospinal tract
      Vestibulo-thalamocortical fibers
    - - Thalamus: Connections with vestibular cortex & reticular formation- *helps in arousal and conscious awareness of the body; helps in discriminating between self movement vs. environment*
      -Vestibular cortex: *at the junction of parietal and insular lobe* *These are targets for afferents along with the cerebellum; both process vestibular information with somatosensory and visual input.*

- **VI. Meiner's Disease**
  - An inner ear disease associated with increase in endolymphatic pressure
  - Characterised by
    - tinnitus
    - vertigo
    - hearing loss
    - vomiting

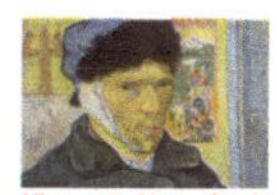

Vincent Van Gogh cut off his ear due to tinnitus from Meniere's disease

On December 23, 1888, Vincent Van Gogh, the legendary French painter, cut off his own ear. A local physician, Dr. Felix Ray, examined him that night and wrote that the painter had been 'assailed by auditory hallucinations' and mutilated himself. Van Gogh committed suicide in 1890. Some American neurologists have concluded that the painter's strange attacks of dizziness, nausea and overwhelming tinnitus (ringing in the ears) were due to Meniere's disease.

DC Mathangi

18. Autonomic Nervous System

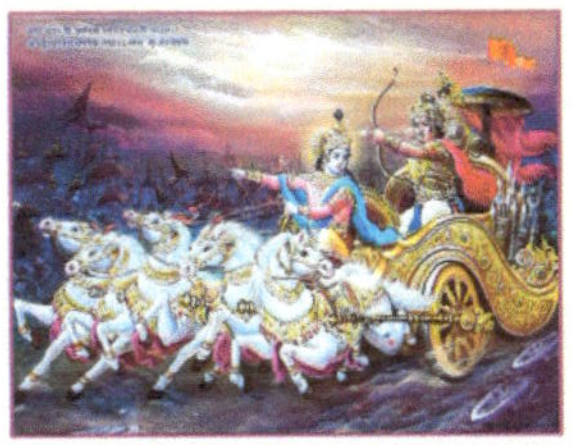

Arjuna, on rising up from his chariot, on realising that he would have to fight his loved ones and relatives tells Bhagwan Krishna *(Gita- Chapter 1, Verse 28-30)*:

Krishna, Krishna
now as I look on
There are my
kinsmen
Arrayed for battle
My mouth is
parching My
hand trembles
My hair stands
upright
My skin burning
The bow Gandiva
slips from my hand
My brain is whirling
Round and round
I can stand no
longer.

Increased activation of the sympathetic nervous system

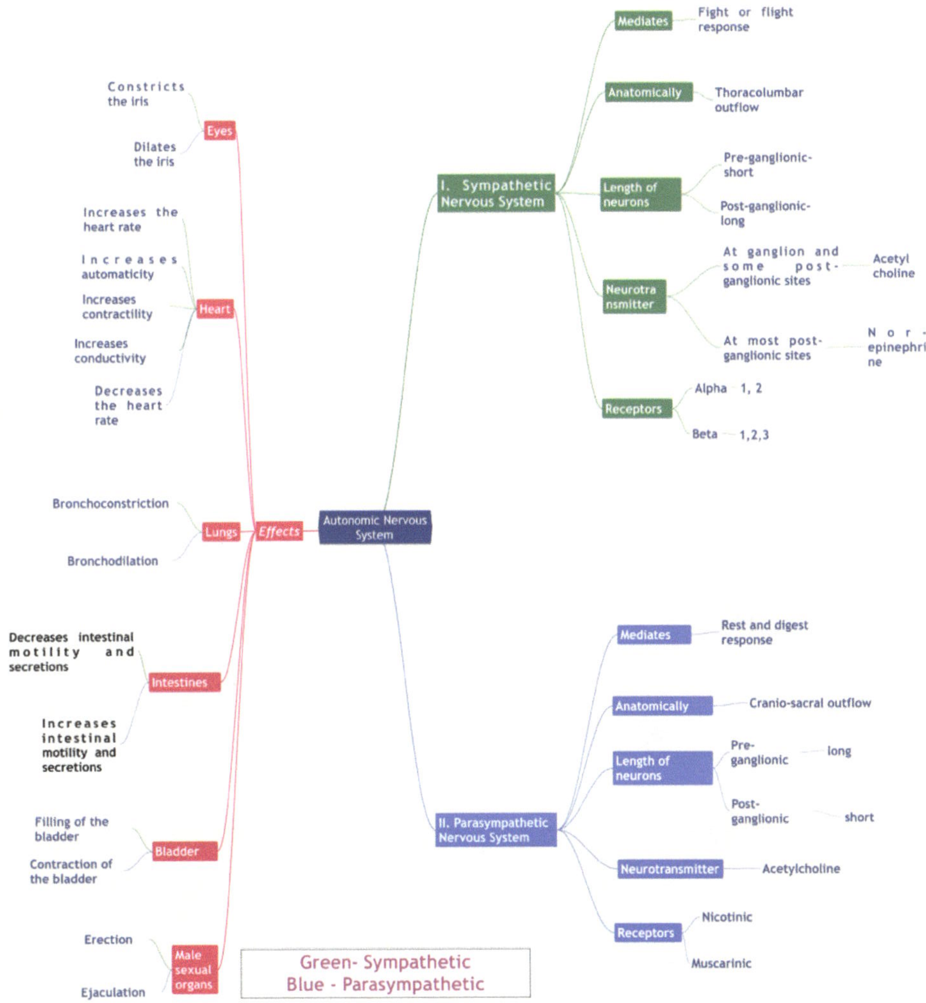

19. Clinical Conditions affecting the Spinal Cord

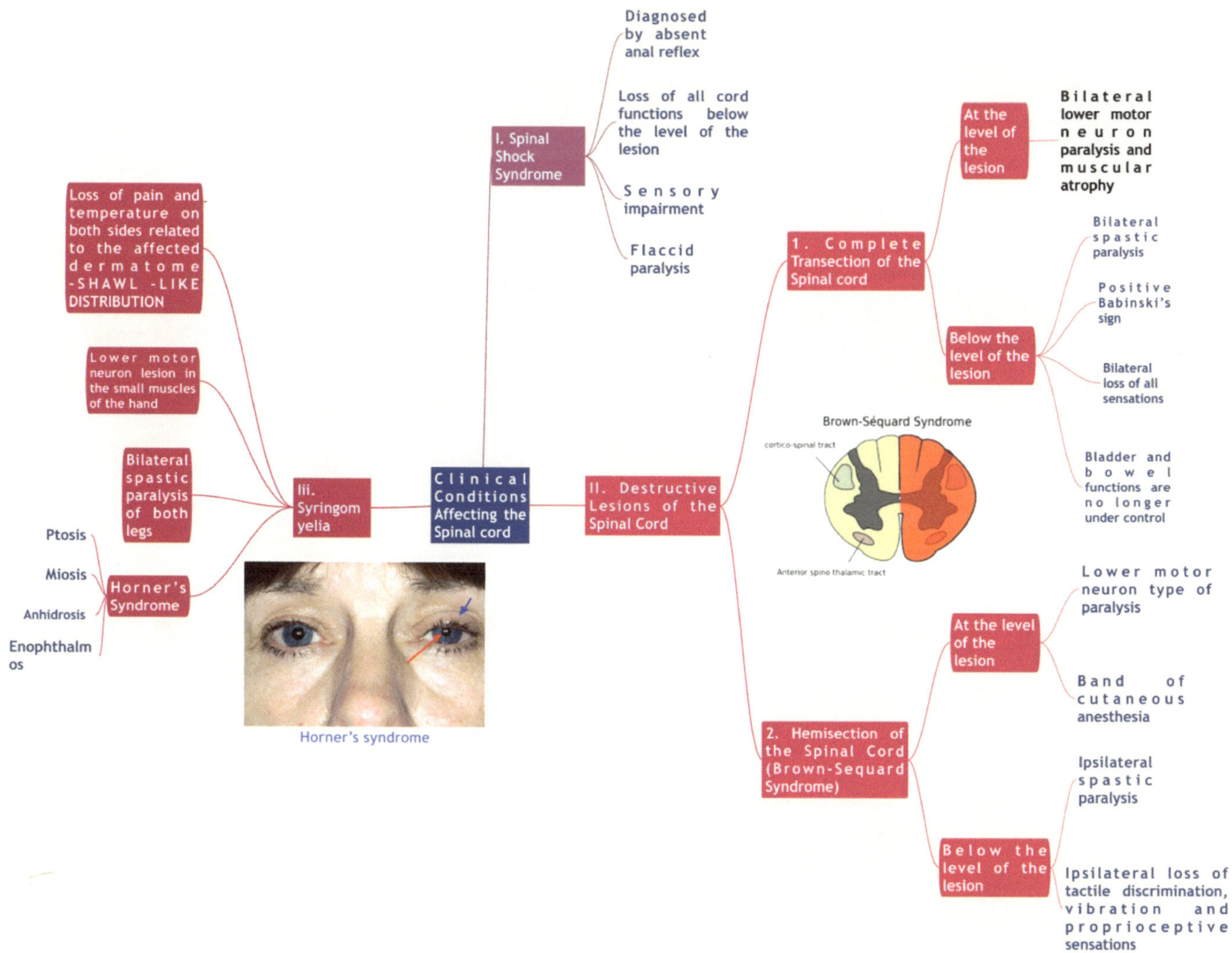

SECTION II

CENTRAL NERVOUS SYSTEM

20. Cerebral Cortex-I

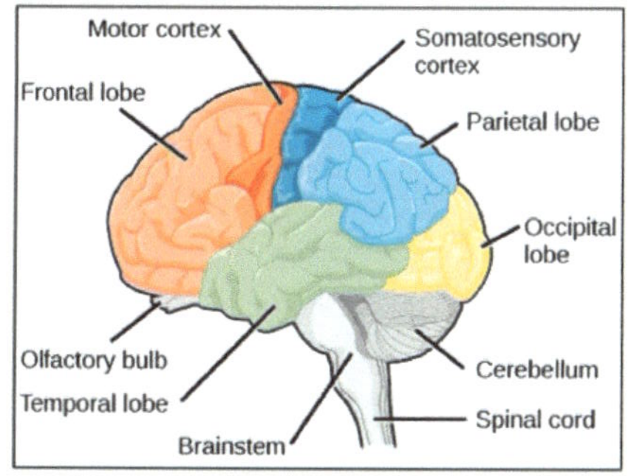

Cerebral Cortex-I

- **I. Frontal Lobe**
  - Area of cortex represented is proportional to the skill involved in performing the movement
  - 1. Primary Motor Area
    - Located in the pre-central gyrus extending into the superior border under the para-central lobule
    - Contains giant pyramidal cells of Betz
    - Inverse representation of the opposite half of the body
  - 2. Secondary Motor Area
    - Middle frontal gyrus of the medial surface
    - Opposite representation of the contra-lateral half of the body
    - Lesions- No loss of movement
  - 3. Frontal eye field Area
    - Middle frontal gyrus
    - Conjugate deviation of the eyes to the opposite side
- **II. Parietal Lobe**
  - 1. Primary Somaesthetic Area
    - Situated in
      - Post-central gyrus on the lateral surface and posterior part of the superior temporal gyrus on the medial surface
    - Characteristics
      - Opposite side of the body is represented as inverted
      - Face, limbs, thumb and index finger have large areas
  - 2. Secondary Somaesthetic Area
    - Superior lip of the posterior limb of the lateral sulcus
    - Functional significance of the part is not understood
  - 3. Somesthetic Association Area
    - Superior parietal lobule extending into the medial surface of the hemisphere
    - Receives and integrates different modalities in the light of past experience

21. Cerebral Cortex-II

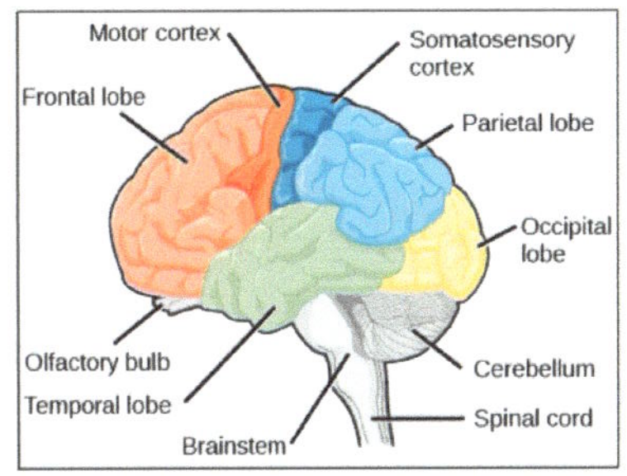

Cerebral Cortex-II

- **III. Temporal Lobe**
  - 1. Primary Auditory Area
    - Situated in the inferior part of the lateral sulcus; includes the gyrus of Heschl
    - Anterior part
      - Recognition of sounds of low intensity
    - Posterior part
      - Recognition of sounds of high intensity
  - 2. Secondary Auditory Area
    - Situated posterior to the primary auditory area in the temporal cortex and posterior part of the superior temporal gyrus on the medial surface
    - Concerned with the integration of various sounds
- **IV. Occipital Lobe**
  - 1. Primary Visual Area
    - Situated in the posterior part of the calcimine sulcus and extends into the occipital lobe
    - Receives afferents from the lateral geniculate body
      - Temporal half of the ipsilateral retina
      - Nasal half of the contralateral retina
    - Superior part of the retina is represented in the superior part of the calcimine sulcus and vice Versa
    - MACULA LUTEA
      - Posterior part of Area 17 and includes 1/3rd of the visual cortex
  - 2. Secondary Visual Area
    - Surrounds the primary visual area on the medial and lateral surface of the hemispheres
    - Receives inputs from Area 17 and other cortical areas and the thalamus
    - Relates the visual information received by the primary visual area to the past visual experience
  - 3. Occipital Eye Field Area
    - Produces conjugate deviation of the eyes to the opposite side
      - Lies in the secondary visual area in humans

Swapnil Paralikar

22. Cerebral Cortex-III

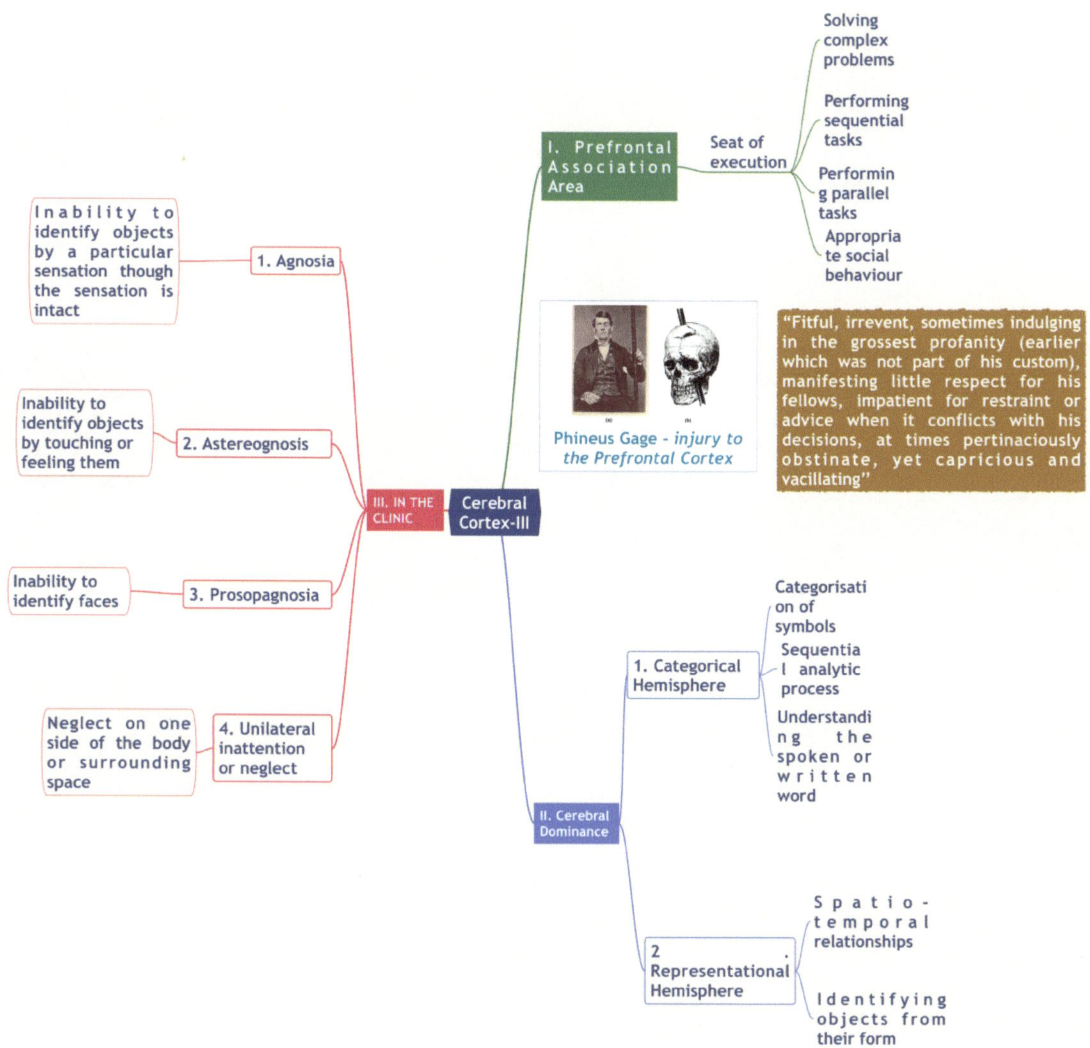

Swapnil Paralikar

23. Thalamus

- **Thalamus**
  - **I. Functional Anatomy**
    - 1. Epithalamus — Pineal gland
    - 2. Thalamus
    - 3. Sub-thalamus — Part of basal ganglia
    - 4. Hypothalamus
  - **II. Organization of thalamic nuclei** — Separated by internal medullary lamina
    - 1. Anterior — Anterior nucleus
    - 2. Medial — Dorsomedian nucleus
    - 3. Lateral
      - Ventro-anterior and Ventro-lateral
      - Ventral postero-medial (VPM) and Ventral postero-lateral (VPL)
      - Pulvinar, Medial Geniculate Body, Lateral Geniculate Body
    - 4. Intra-laminar
    - 5. Lateral reticular nucleus
  - **III. Connections of thalamic nuclei**
    - 1. Relay nuclei
      - Basal Ganglia and Cerebellum → Ventro-anterior and Ventro-lateral nucleus → Cerebral Cortex
      - Medial Lemniscus, Spino-thalamic Tract → Ventral postero-lateral (VPL) → Somato-sensory Cortex
      - Medial Lemniscus, Spino-thalamic Tract (face area) → Ventral postero-medial (VPM) → Somato-sensory Cortex
      - Brachium of inferior colliculus → Medial geniculate body → Auditory Cortex
      - Optic Tract → Lateral geniculate body → Optic Tract
    - 2. Association nuclei
      - Dorso-median nucleus — Pre-frontal Cortex
      - Pulvinar — Parieto-temporo-occipital cortex
    - 3. Lateral reticular nucleus — Projects GABAergic projection to other thalamic inputs

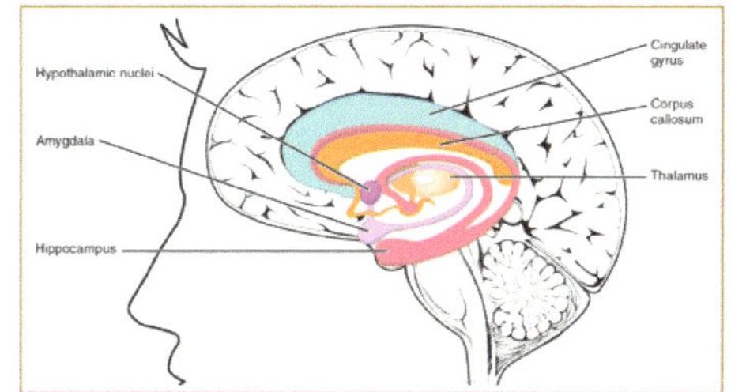

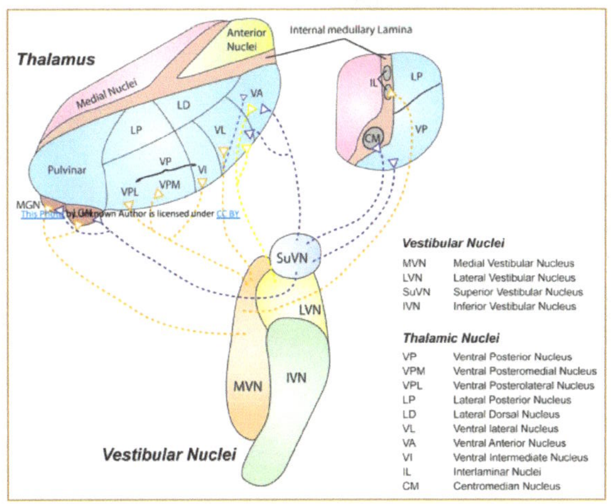

Swapnil Paralikar

24. Functions of Hypothalamus

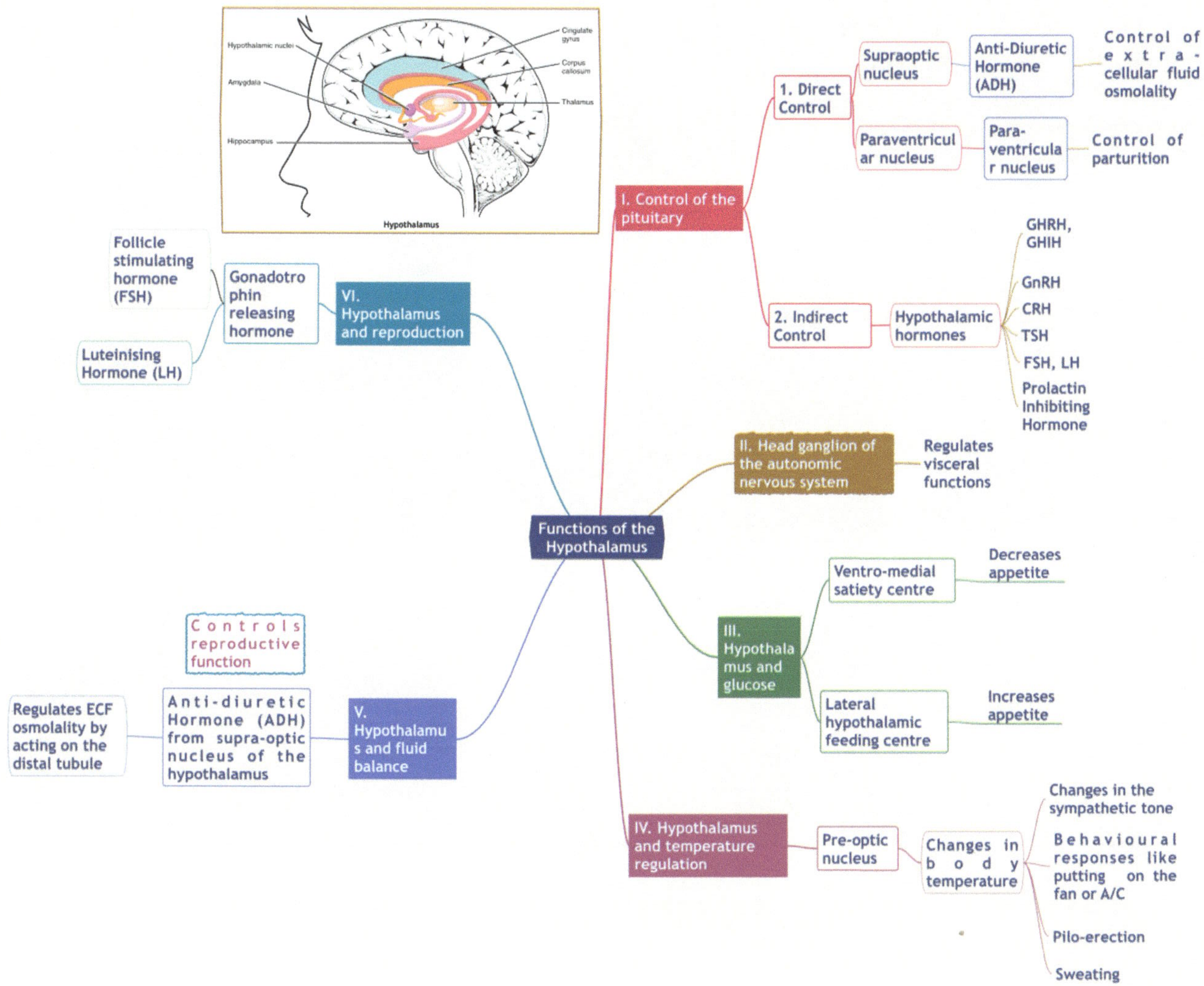

Swapnil Paralikar

25. Basal Ganglia

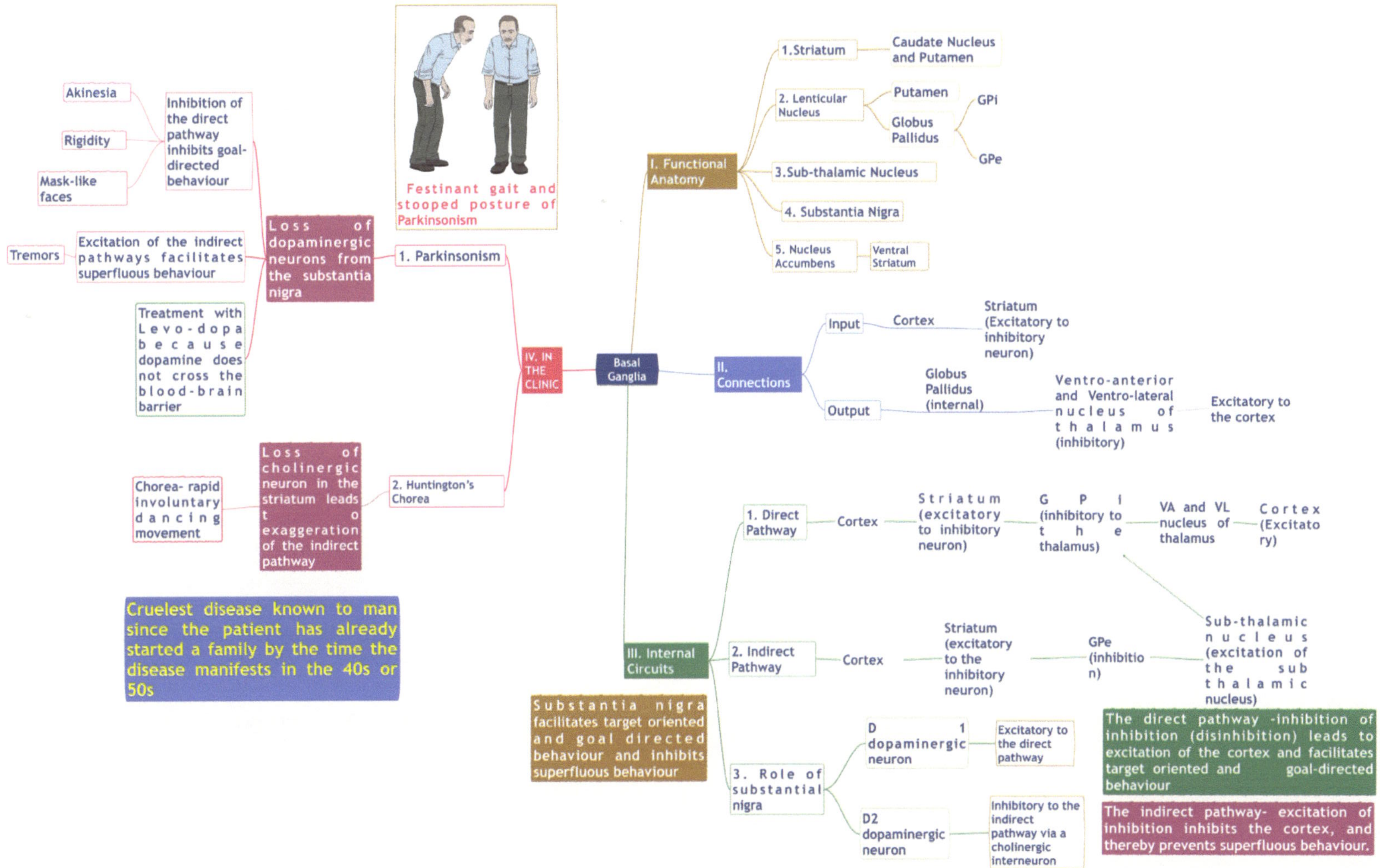

Swapnil Paralikar

26. Cerebellum- I-Introduction, Connections and Functions

- CEREBELLUM-I
  - I. Divisions
    - Physiologically
      - Vestibulo-cerebellum
      - Spino-cerebellum
      - Cerebro-cerebellum

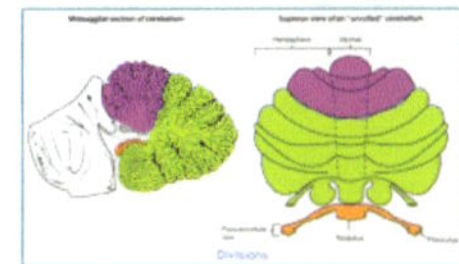

  - II. Histologically
    - 1. Layers
      - Molecular layer — Basket and stellate cells
      - Purkinge cell layer
      - Granule cell layer — Granule and Golgi cells
    - 2. Fibers
      - Climbing Fibres — Fibres from the inferior olive
      - Mossy Fibres — All the other afferent inputs into the cerebellum

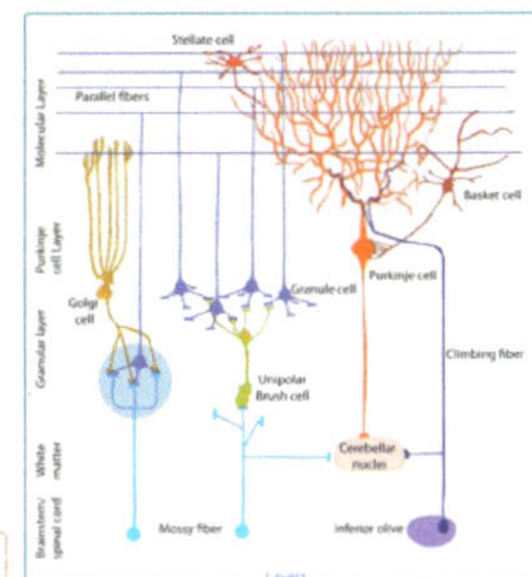

  - III.A. Connections and Functions
    - 1. Vestibulo-cerebellum
      - Connections — With vestibular apparatus
      - Functions — Maintenance of tone, posture and equilibrium
  - III.B. Connections and Functions
    - 1. Spinocerebellum
      - Connections
        - Afferent — Dorsal and ventral spino-cerebellar tract
        - Efferent — Cerebello-olivary tract
      - Functions
        - Helps in smooth, co-ordinating movements of muscles
        - Helps in ballistic movements through effects on rate, range, force and direction of movement
      - Effects of damage
        - Rapidly and difficulty in initiating movements
        - Cerebellar ataxia
    - 3. Cerebro-cerebellum
      - Connections
        - Afferent
          - Olivo-cerebellar tract
          - Ponto-cerebellar tract
        - Efferent
          - Dentato-thalamic tract
          - Dentato-rubral tract
      - Functions
        - Planning of sequential movements
        - Timing of complex movements
        - Extra-motor prediction of motor function
      - Effects of damage
        - Ataxia, Asynergia, hypotonia, timing defect

DC Mathangi

27. Cerebellum- In the Clinic

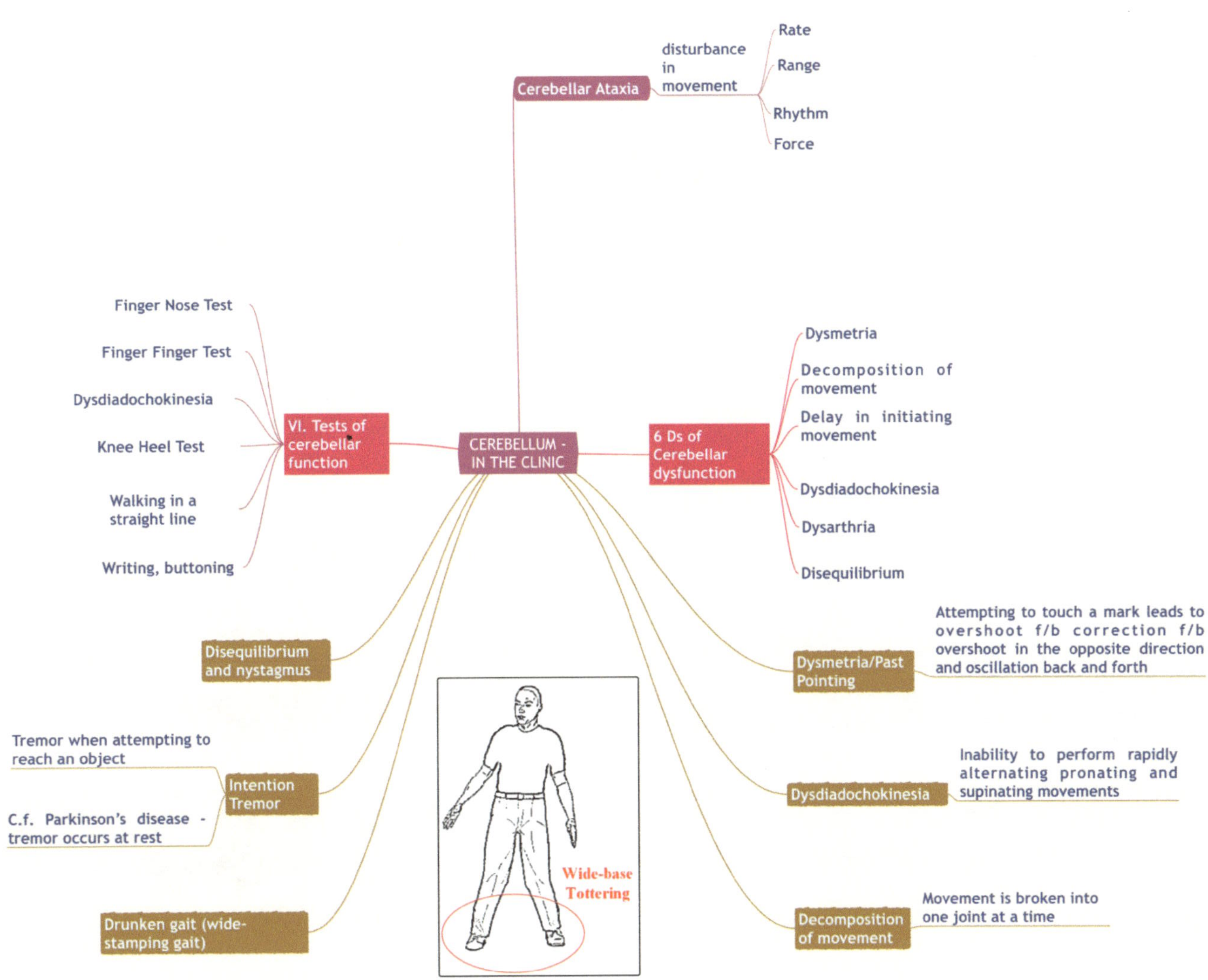

Swapnil Paralikar

28.Limbic System

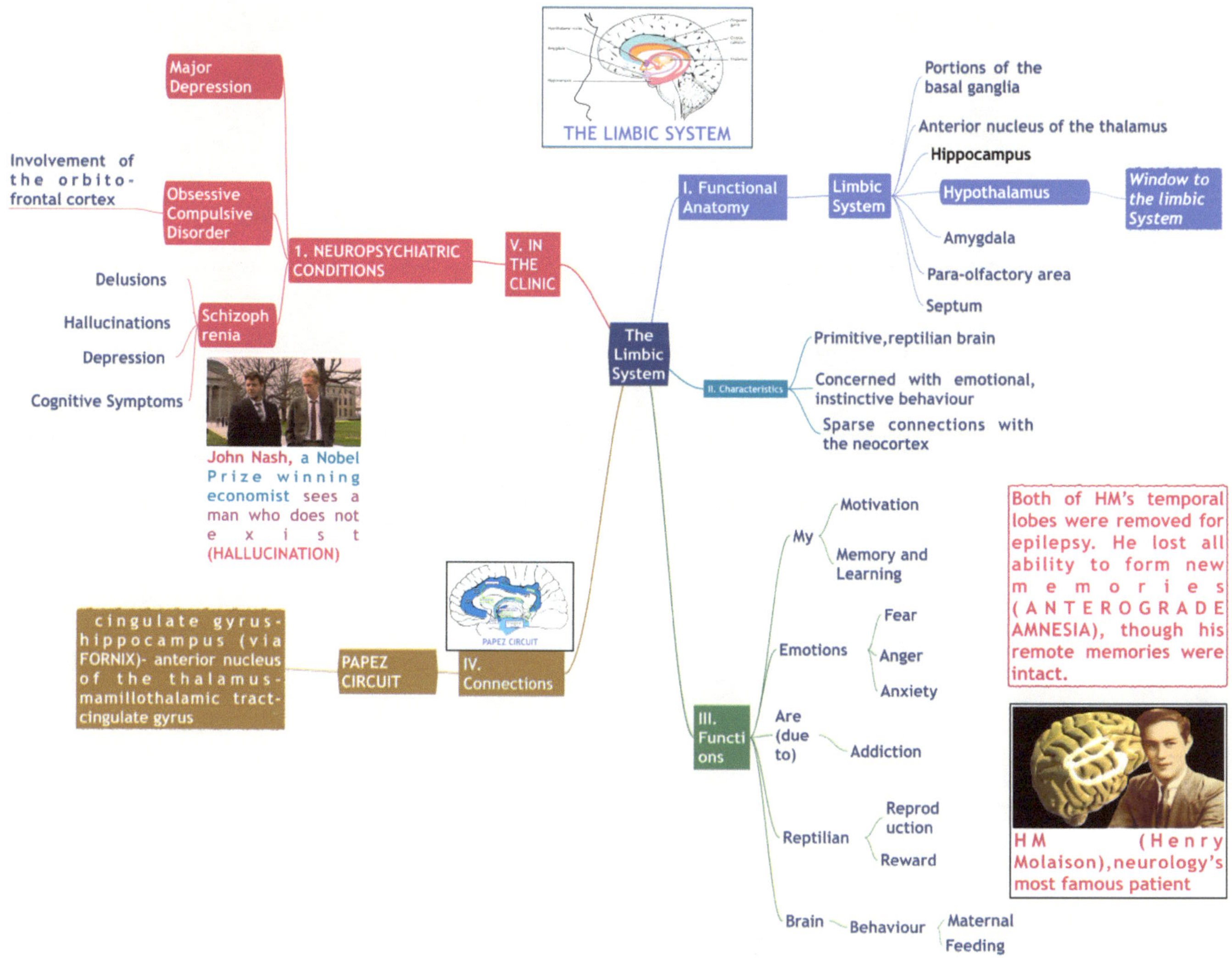

Riituparna Barooah

SECTION III

HIGHER FUNCTIONS

29. Physiology of Sleep

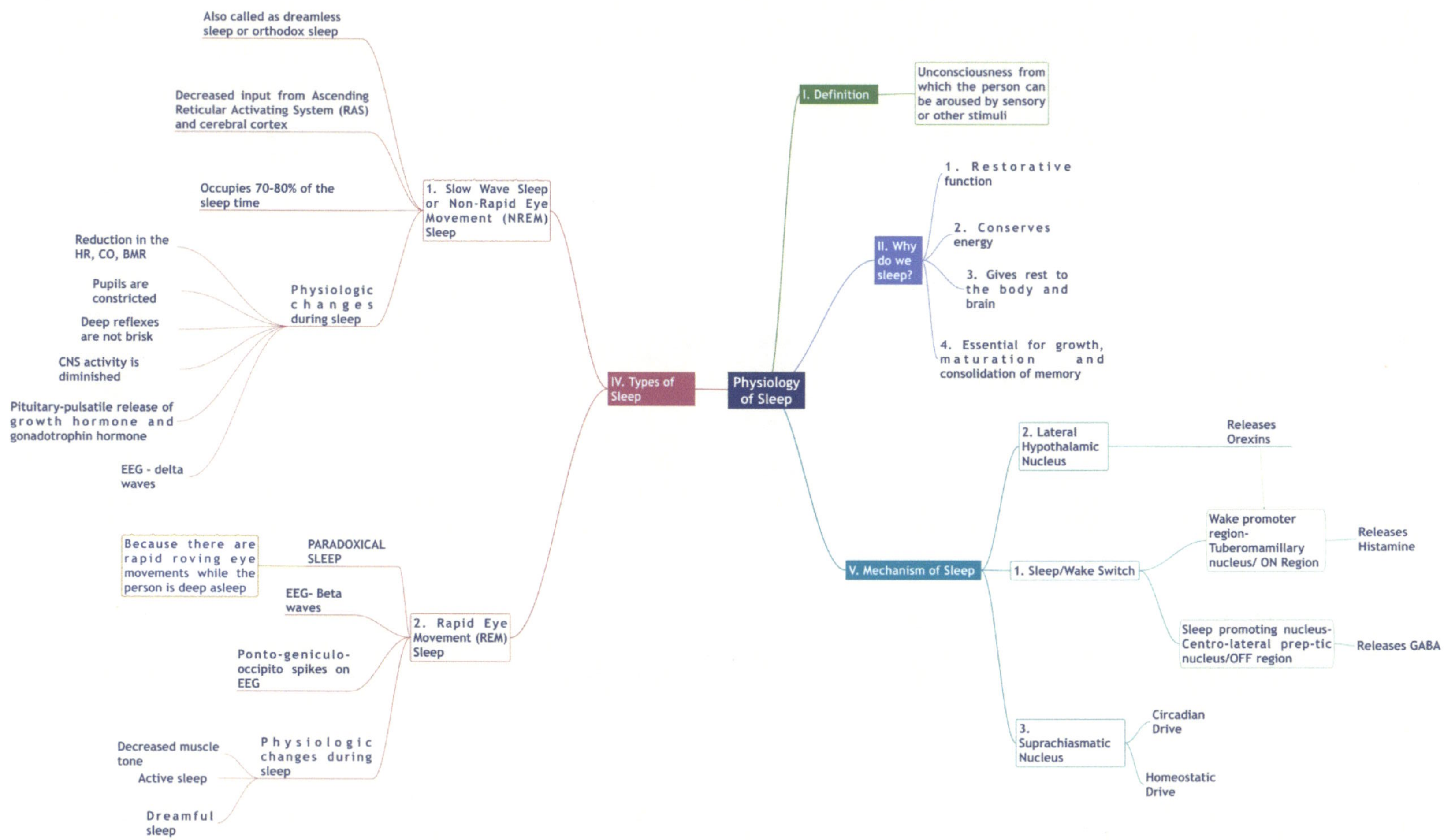

DC Mathangi

30. Disorders of Sleep

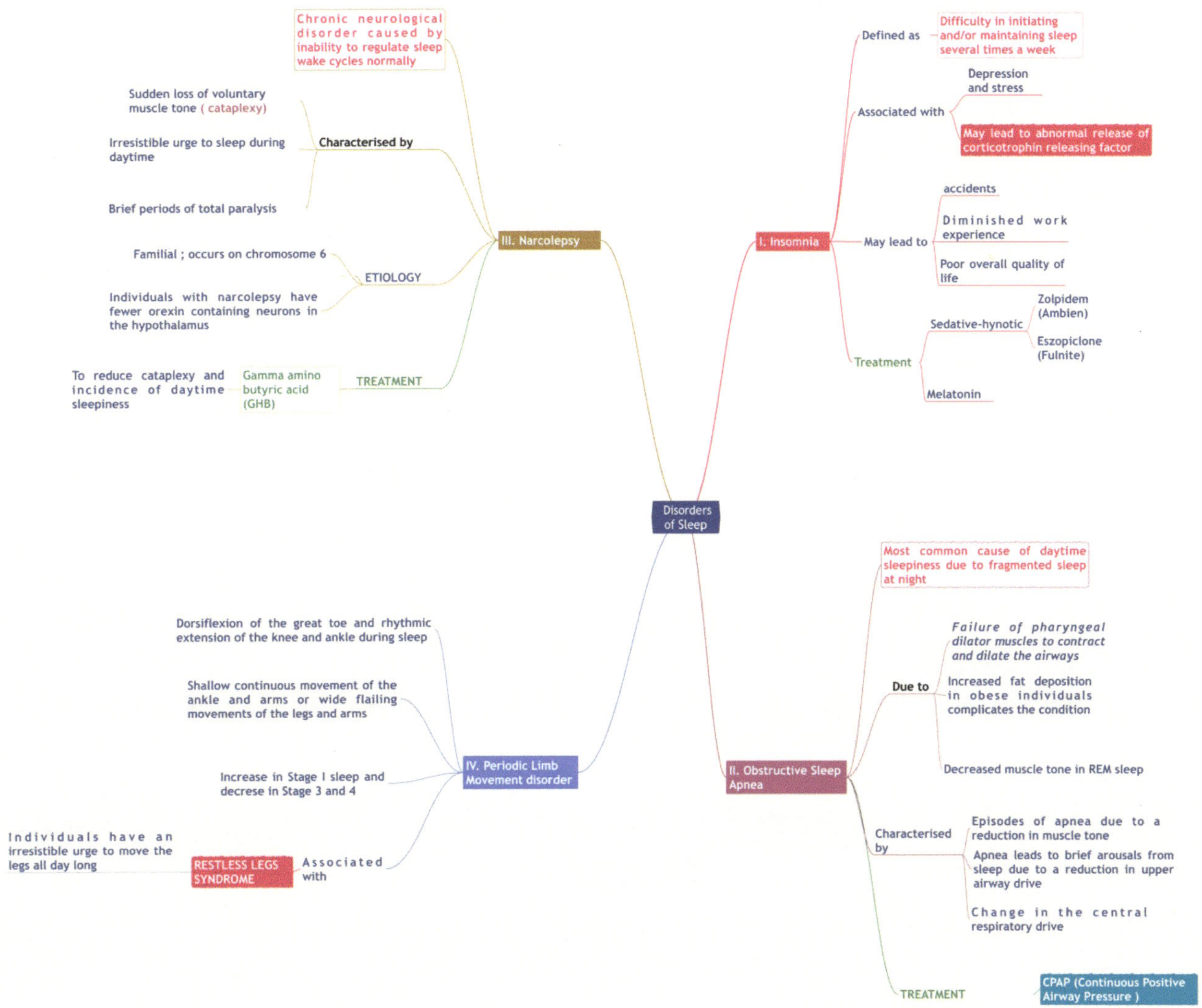

Swapnil Paralikar

31. Electro-encephalogram

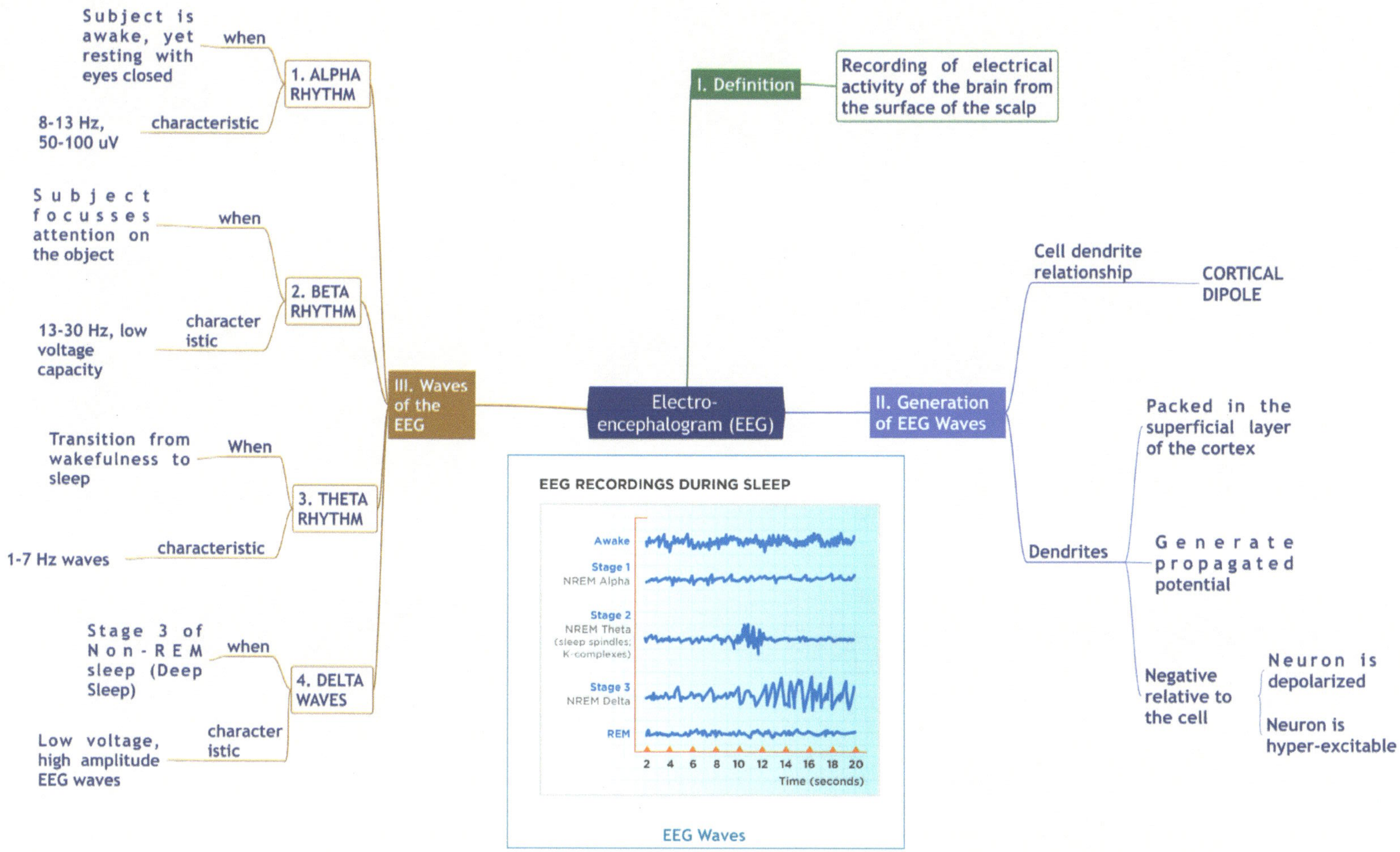

Swapnil Paralikar

32. Learning and Memory

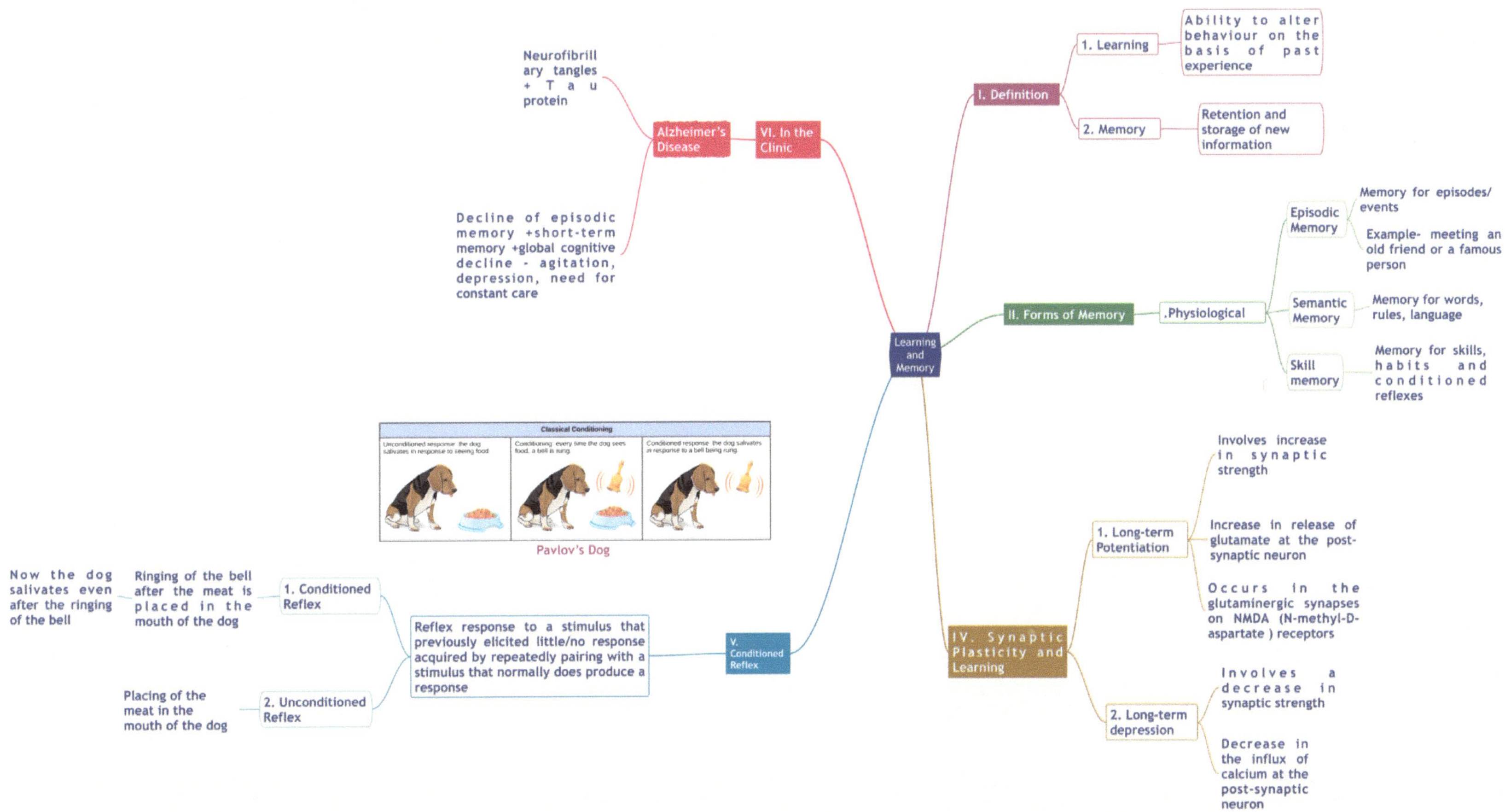

Swapnil Paralikar

33. Aphasias

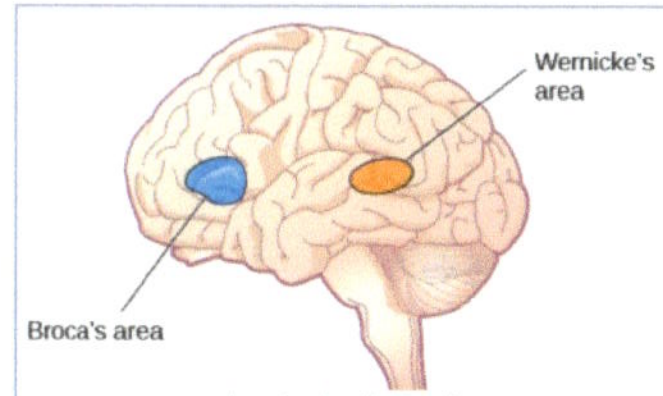

Areas involved in Speech

Aphasias

Aphasias are disorders of speech or language that are not due to visual or hearing or mental probelms

- **I. Wernicke's Aphasia**
  - Wernicke's area is located at the temporo-parieto-occipital junction; *helps in understanding the written and oral words*
  - Patient cannot understand the written or oral word
  - Speech is full of jargon and neologisms that makes little sense
  - Neologisms - using the word 'book' instead of a 'pen' ; Using the word 'flig' instead of 'flag'
  - Paraphrasia- I want to eat an 'apple' instead of I want to eat a 'banana'
- **II. Broca's Aphasia**
  - Broca's area converts the understanding gained in the Wernicke's area into a detailed and co-ordinated pattern of vocalisation
  - Patient is unable to conjure up words
  - Speech may be limited to two or three words which he may be speaking at the time of trauma or accident
- **III. Anomic Aphasia**
  - Trouble understanding the written language or pictures due to lesion in the ANGULAR GYRUS of the categorical hemisphere
- **IV. Global Aphasia**
  - Areas of temporal, parietal and occipital cortex that support the knowledge of words and their meaning
    - Word Salad- meaningless, voluminous speech
  - Areas of frontal lobe that permit sentence level processing
    - Errors of syntax and sentence formation
- ***Stuttering***
  - RIGHT CEREBRAL DOMINANCE & widespread increase in the activity in the cerebral cortex and cerebellum

Swapnil Paralikar

34. Neurotransmitters-I

Neurotransmitters-I

- **I. Acetylcholine**
  - The first neurotransmitter to be discovered
  - 1. Site of action
    - all the neutrons which exit the CNS
      - Pre-ganglionic autonomic neurons
      - Post-ganglionic parasympathetic neurons
      - Post-ganglionic sympathetic neurons innervating sweat glands
      - Neuro-muscular Junction
  - 2. Receptors
    - 1. Nicotinic
      - Neuronal at the autonomic ganglia
      - Muscular at the Neuro-muscular junction
    - 2. Muscarinic
      - M1 and M5 in the CNS
      - M2 in the heart
      - M3 and M4 in the glands
  - 3. In the Clinic
    - Botulinum Toxin (BOTOX) injection
      - Prevents the release of Acetylcholine
        - Prevents wrinkles
        - Relieves oesophageal spasm
- **II. Dopamine= movement**
  - 1. Nigrostrial System
    - Excitatory to the direct pathway via D1 dopaminergic receptors
    - Inhibitory to the indirect pathway via D2 dopaminergic receptors
    - Loss of these dopaminergic neurons leads to Parkinsonism
    - It is treated with Levo-dopa because dopamine does not cross the blood-brain barrier
  - 2. Meso-limbic System
    - From the ventral tegmentum to the nucleus accumbens in the midbrain
      - reward
      - addiction
        - alcohol
        - Smoking
        - Compulsive and habitual need for a substance inspite of negative health consequences
  - 3. Meso-cortical system
    - From the ventral tegmentum to the pre-frontal cortex
      - Implicated in schizophrenia
        - hallucinations
        - delusions

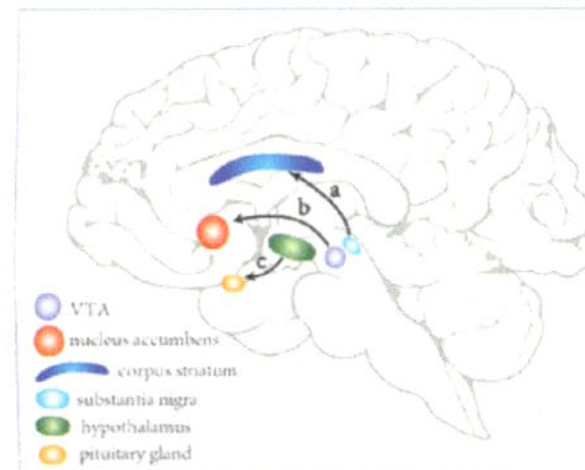

Dopamine pathways in the brain

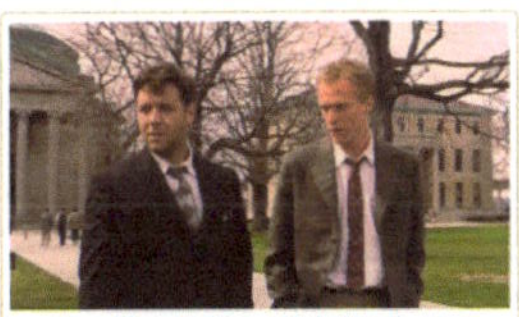

The film 'A Beautiful Mind' *-the protagonist Jon Nash (Russel Crowe) talks to a man who does not exist-* VISUAL HALLUCINATION

Swapnil Paralikar

35. Neurotransmitters-II

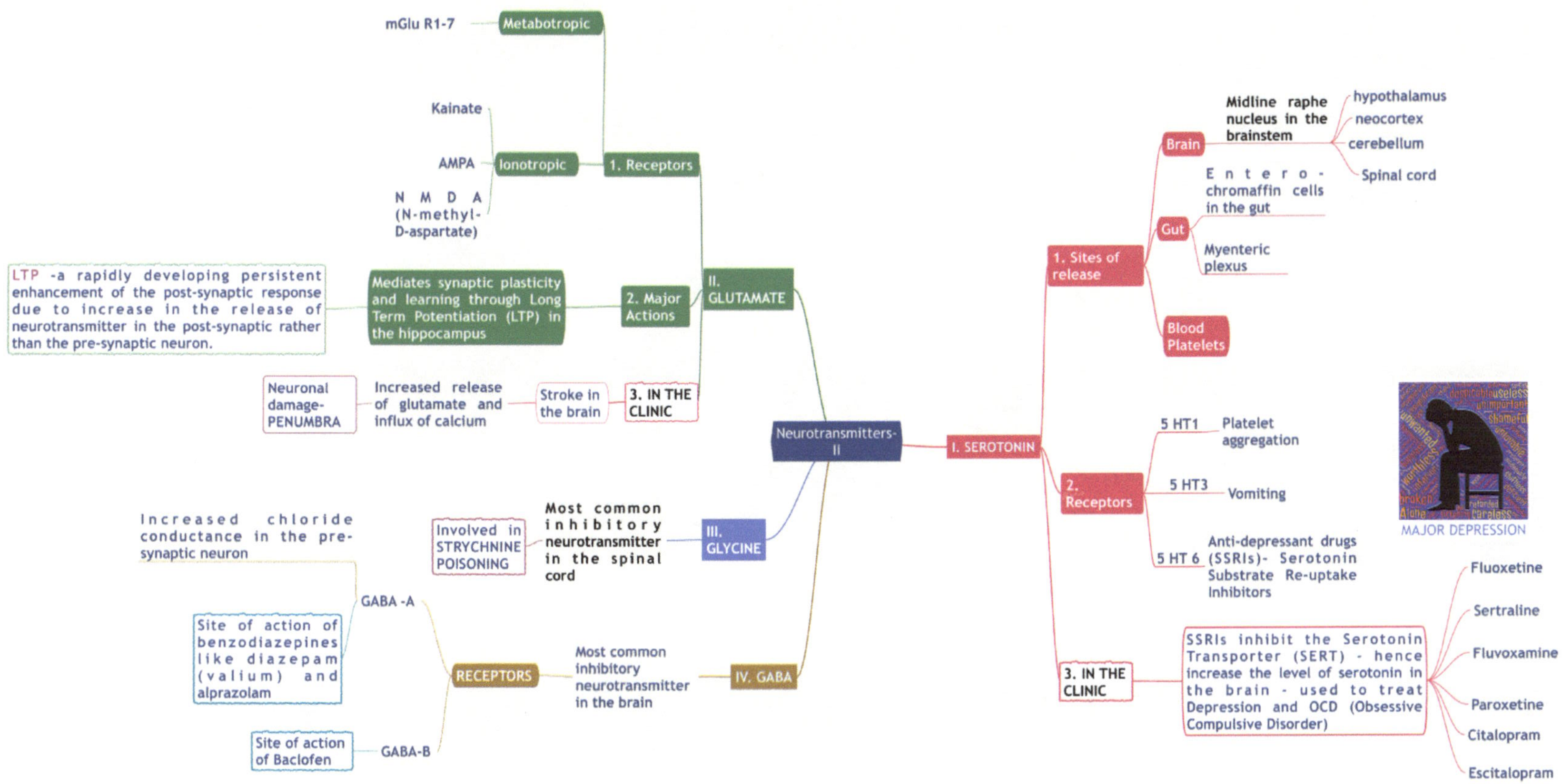

Swapnil Paralikar

SECTION IV

SPECIAL SENSES

36. Physiology of Taste Sensation

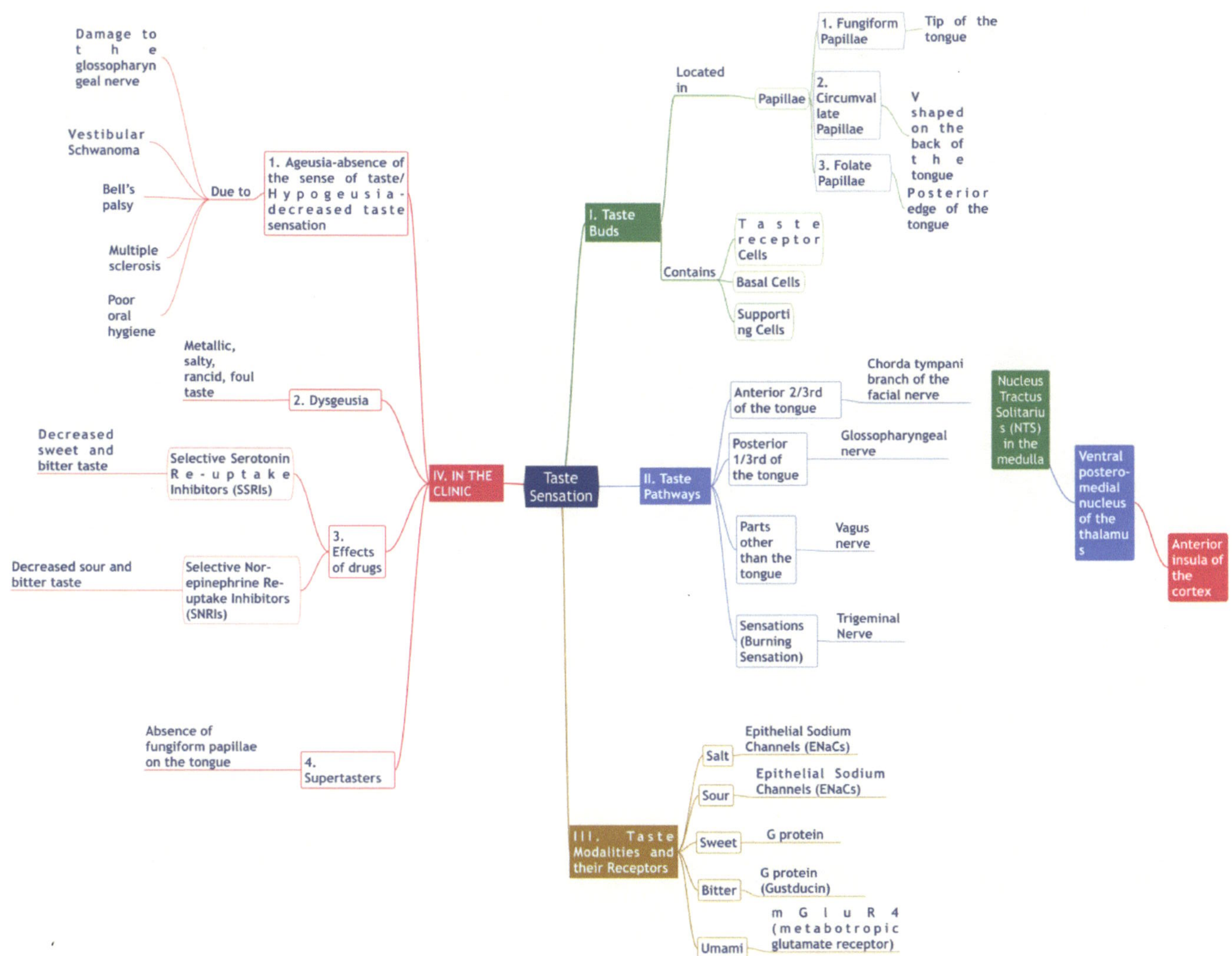

Swapnil Paralikar

37. Physiology of Olfaction

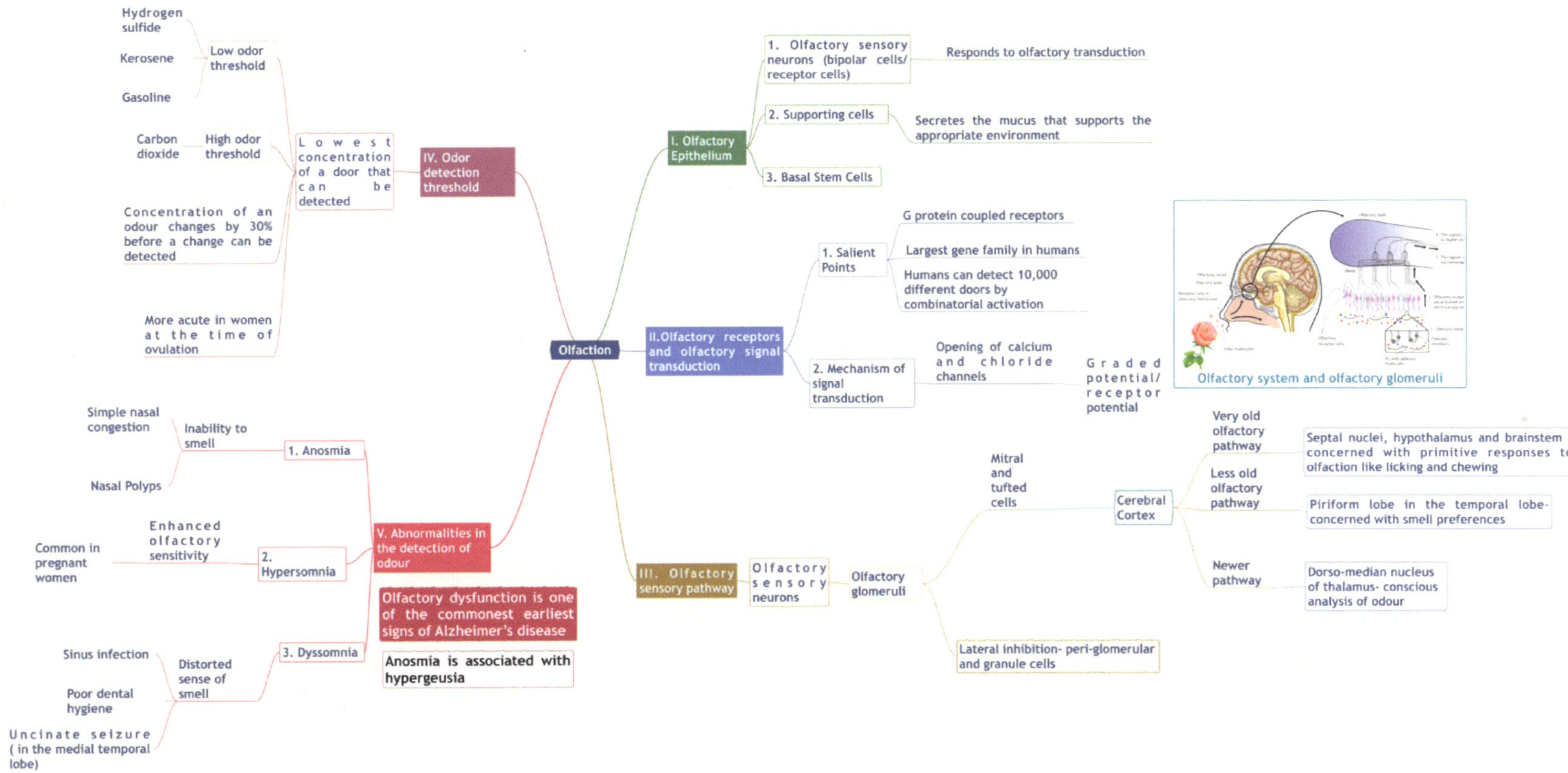

Swapnil Paralikar

38. Physiology of Hearing-I

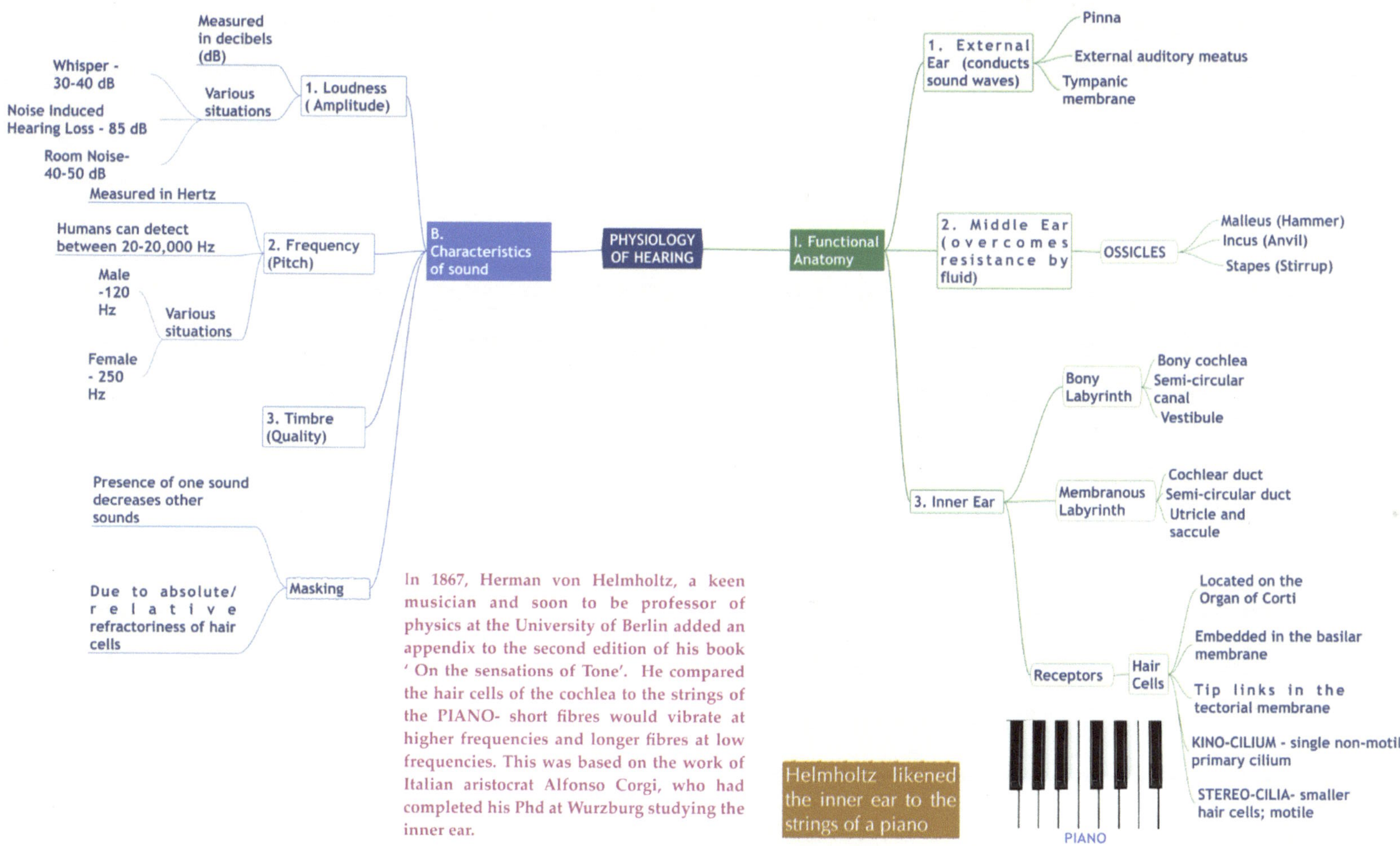

In 1867, Herman von Helmholtz, a keen musician and soon to be professor of physics at the University of Berlin added an appendix to the second edition of his book ' On the sensations of Tone'. He compared the hair cells of the cochlea to the strings of the PIANO- short fibres would vibrate at higher frequencies and longer fibres at low frequencies. This was based on the work of Italian aristocrat Alfonso Corgi, who had completed his Phd at Wurzburg studying the inner ear.

Helmholtz likened the inner ear to the strings of a piano

Thejaswini KO

39. Physiology of Hearing-II-Auditory Pathway

AUDITORY PATHWAY

I. From Hair Cells to Cortex

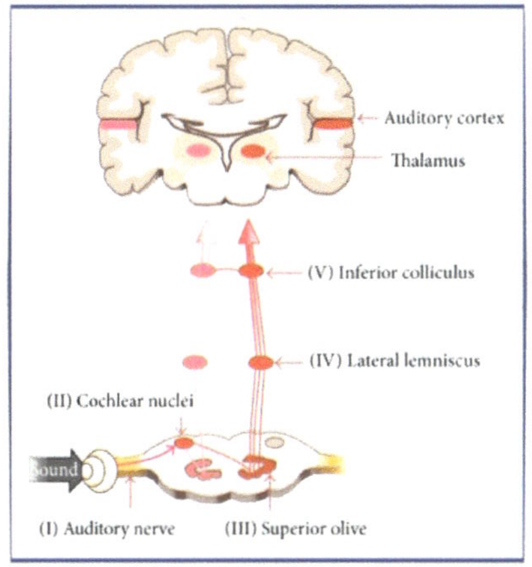

1. Hair cells
2. Auditory nerve
3. Cochlear nerve at the point-medullary junction
4. Via trapezoid body to the superior olivary nucleus
5. Via lateral lemniscus to the inferior colliculi
6. Medial geniculate body of the thalamus
7. Auditory cortex-transverse gyrus on the superior surface of the temporal bone

II. IN THE CLINIC

ACOUSTIC NEUROMA

Auditory nerve lies at the junction of the pons, medulla and cerebellum. Common site of a slow growing tumour acoustic neuroma. Causes pressure on the 7th, 8th and 9th nerves

Hearing loss is the initial symptom followed by tinnitus, vertigo, nystagmus, etc.

Thejaswini KO

40. Hearing Loss

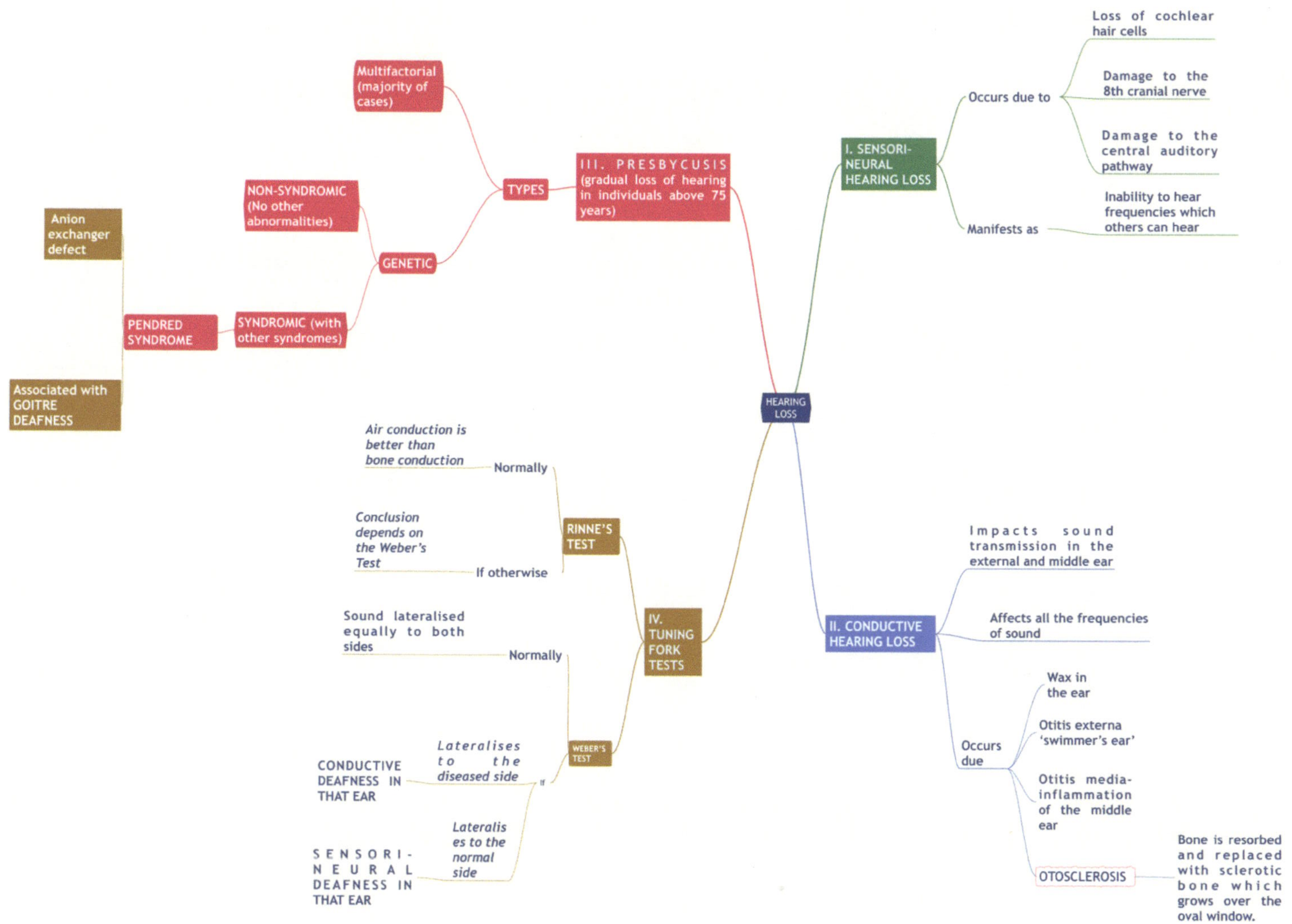

Thejaswini KO and Swapnil Paralikar

41. Errors of Refraction

Errors of Refraction

- **I. The optic arrangement: The eye as a camera**
  - 1. Lens system : Refractive index in the eye a) Anterior surface of the cornea b) Posterior surface of the cornea c) Anterior surface of the lens d) Posterior surface of the lens
  - 2. Aperture system: Pupil
  - 3. Film: Retina
- **II. The process of Image formation (Image of Reduced eye)**
  - 1. Refraction : Depends on the type of lens a) Convex lens: Light rays converge b) Concave lens: Light rays diverge c) Cylindrical lens: unlike spherical lens all light rays come to focal line rather than focal point
  - 2. Focus : Depends on the refractive power of the lens system a) measured in diopters b) 1 diopter : 1/ principal focus of the lens
    - Power of human eye is 60 diopter a) 2/3rd by anterior surface of cornea b) 1/3rd by crystalline lens
  - 3. Image: real and inverted on retina
- **III. Mechanism for altering focus**
  - 1. Changing refractive power of lens: *Accommodation reflex*
    - At rest: a) ciliary body relaxed b) suspensory ligament is tense c) lens flattened or less curved
    - When focussing near object: a) ciliary body contracts b) suspensory ligament is relaxed c) lens become more curved
  - 2. Changing Pupillary Aperture : Changing depth of focus
    - 1. Smaller pupillary aperture : Larger depth of focus
    - 2. Larger pupillary aperture : Smaller depth of focus
- **IV. Defects of optical system**
  - 1. Errors of refraction
    - 1. *Myopia (Nearsightedness)* : - Focus in front of retina -Eyeball too long/ lens system too weak -Corrected by: CONCAVE LENS (which diverge light rays)
    - 2. *Hyperopia (Far sightedness)* : Focus behind retina -Eyeball too short, lens system too strong -Correction: Convex Lens (which converge light rays)
    - 3. Astigmatism -Focus at different points - Non-uniform curvature of cornea -Correction: Cylindrical Lens
  - 2. Defects in accomodation
    - Presbyopia : -Lens loses capacity to change curvature/ loss of accomodation -Occurs due to loss of elasticity of lens capsule -Corrected by convex lens

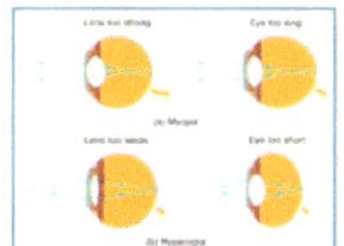

Errors of Refraction

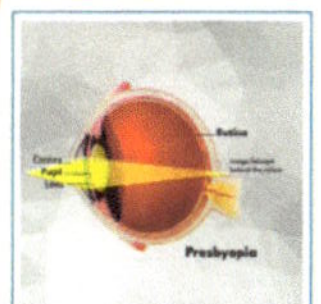

Presbyopia

Madhulika Monga

42. Glaucoma

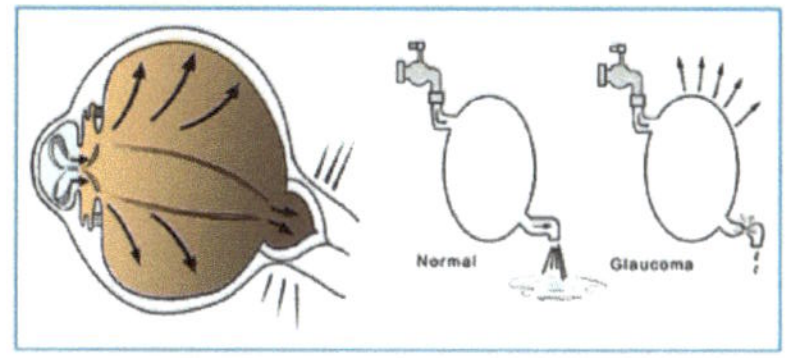

GLAUCOMA

- **I. FUNCTIONAL ANATOMY**
  - 1. Anterior Chamber
    - Bounded anteriorly by the posterior surface of the retina — Bounded posteriorly by the anterior surface of the lens
  - 2. Posterior Chamber
    - Bounded anteriorly by the posterior surface of the iris — Bounded posteriorly by the anterior surface of the lens
  - 3. Choroid
  - 4. Aqueous Humour
    - Ultra-filtrate of plasma
    - Formed by ciliary processes
    - Protein free and rich in ascorbic acid
  - 5. OPTIC DISC
    - 3 mm medial and above the posterior pole of the eye
    - Appears white in fundoscopy-AVASCULAR
    - Ganglion cells fibres and central retinal vein enters the eye
  - 6. FUNDUS
    - Posterior portion of the interior of the eye
    - Red background due to choroid vessels
    - Arterioles are readily visible
- **II. DEFINITION**
  - Damage to the retinal ganglion cells
  - Increased Intra-ocular pressure is JUST A SYMPTOM OF GLAUCOMA(Normal Intra-ocular Pressure is 12-20 mmHg)
- **III. TYPES AND CLASSIFICATION**
  - 1. Congenital and developmental
    - Developmental anomalies of the angle of anterior chamber
  - 2. Primary Glaucoma
    - Without any obvious ocular or systemic cause
    - Occurs commonly after 40 years
    - Closure of angle of anterior chamber
  - 3. Secondary Glaucoma
    - Rise in intra-ocular pressure due to systemic or ocular cause
- **IV. DIAGNOSIS**
  - Tonometry
  - Perimetry
  - Fundoscopy
- **V. CLINICAL FEATURES**
  - Rainbow halos
  - Pain behind the eyes
  - Hardened eyes
  - Restriction of field of vision
  - Gradual loss of vision
  - Watering of the affected eye

Rituparna Barooah

43. Retina

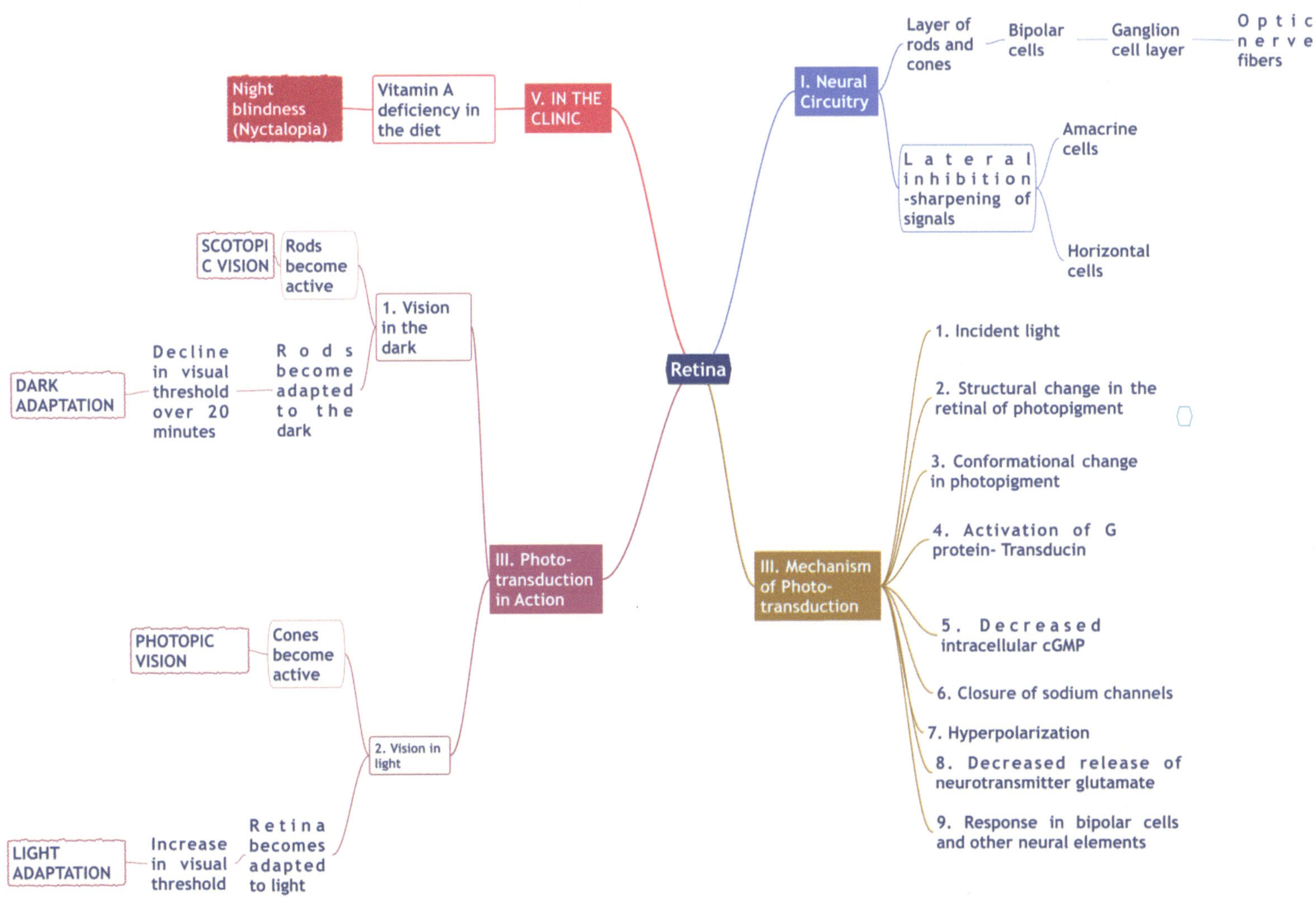

Swapnil Paralikar

44. Color Vision

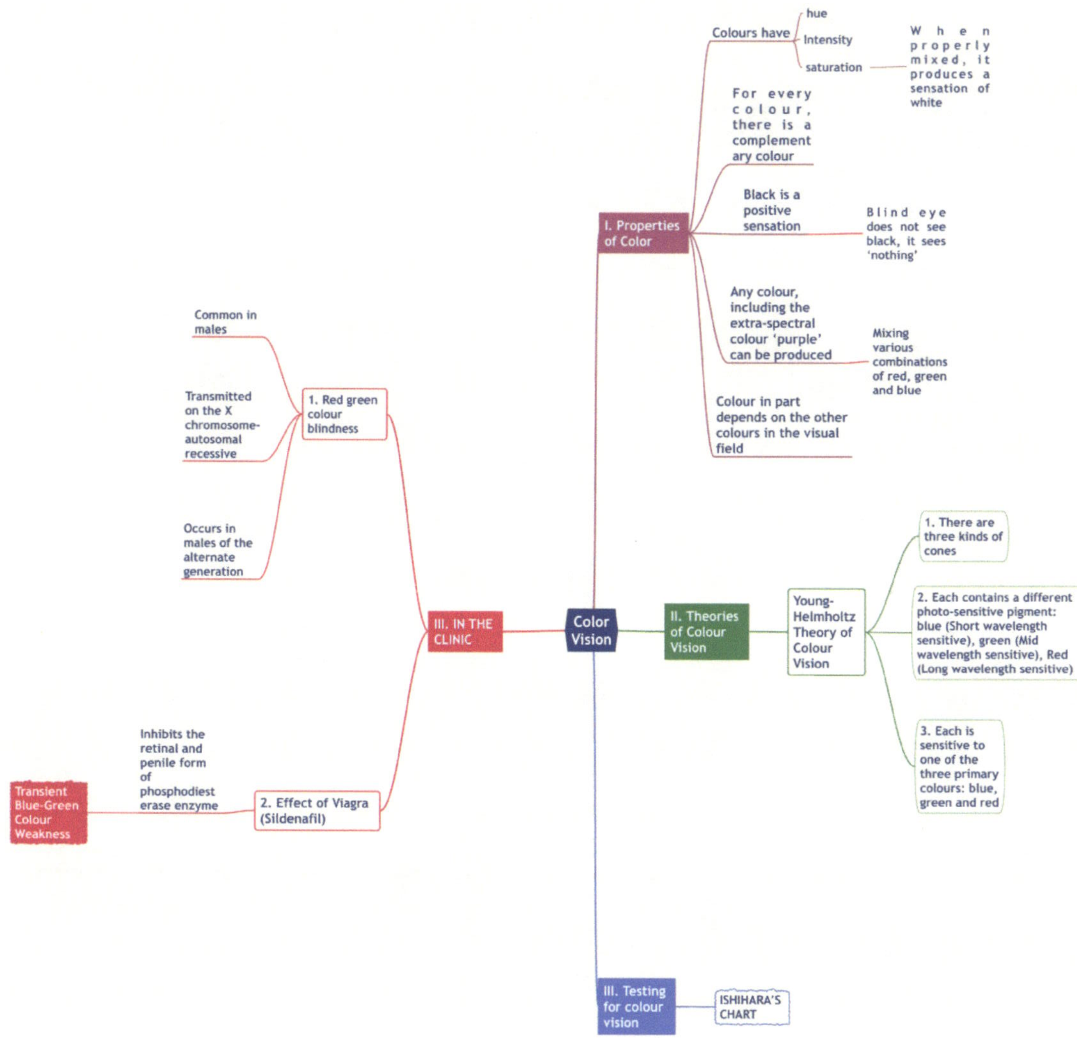

Swapnil Paralikar

45. Optic Pathway and its lesions

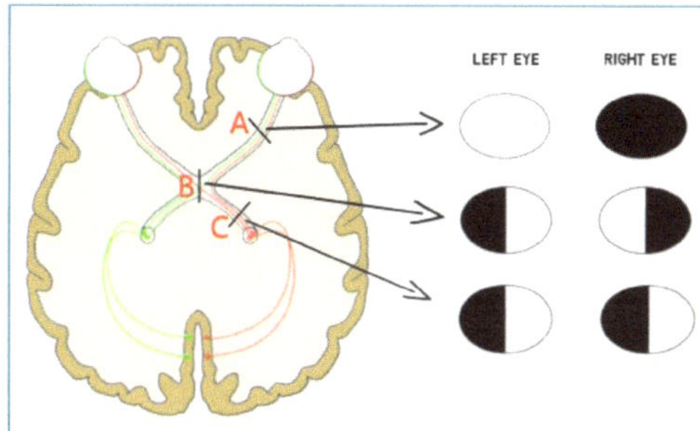

Visual Pathway and its lesions

Visual Pathway

- **I. Visual Pathway**
  - Photoreceptors in the retina
  - Optic nerve nasal fibres- Temporal field of vision; Optic nerve temporal fibres- nasal field of vision
  - Crossing of nasal fibres at optic chiasma-Optic radiation
  - Primary visual cortex- Area 17
  - Secondary visual cortex- Area 18
- **II. Lesions and their effects**
  - Optic nerve — Total blindness in the ipsilateral eye-ANOPIA (A)
  - Crossed fibres of the optic chiasma — Heternonymous Hemianopia- Bitemporal (B)
  - Uncrossed fibres of the optic chiasma — Homonymous Hemianopia
  - Optic tract — Contra-lateral Hemianopia
  - Optic radiation — Homonymous Hemianopia (C)
  - Visual cortex — Homonymous Hemianopia with macular sparring

DC Mathangi

Two roads diverged in a yellow wood,

And I took the one less travelled by,

And that has made all the difference...

Robert Frost

www.ingramcontent.com/pod-product-compliance
Lightning Source LLC
LaVergne TN
LVHW070955210926
848482LV00002B/219